drkamalkv's classes

LMR MANUAL

For FMGE & NEET-PG

Volume - 1

(Non-clinical Subjects)

Anatomy, Physiology, Biochemistry
Pathology, Pharmacology, Microbiology & Parasitology,
Forensic Medicine & PSM

Kamal KV MBBS MS (Orthopedics)
Ex-Senior Resident: Safdarjung, ESI – Okhla, Fortis – Noida
Ponseti and Ilizarov Techniques Fellow (Akola),
Madhya Pradesh – Indian Orthopedic Association
Hand Surgery Fellow (Pune), Maharashtra, India

PEEPEE PUBLISHERS AND DISTRIBUTORS (P) LTD.®

drkamalkv's classes LMR MANUAL FOR FMGE & NEET-PG

Published by
Pawaninder P. Vij and Anupam Vij

Peepee Publishers and Distributors (P) Ltd.
Head Office: 160, Shakti Vihar, Pitam Pura
Delhi-110034 (India)

Correspondence Address:
7/31, First Floor, Ansari Road, Daryaganj
New Delhi-110002 (India)
Ph: 41512412, 23246245, 9811156083
e-mail: peepee160@yahoo.co.in
e-mail: peepee160@gmail.com
www.peepeepub.com

First Edition: 2019

ISBN : 978-81-8445-271-6

Dedication to

This title is dedicated to all the (past & present) students of **drkamalkv's classes for FMGE & NEET-PG**.

It's their faith and support, which is helping me in surviving this competitive world of coaching.

I teach all the subjects singly and theoretically it is seems very difficult to teach all subjects singly, but the unconditional support and faith of my dear students had made it practically possible.

drkamalkv

Contact:
Cell & WhatsApp: 84 7000 4333
Website: www.**drkamalkvgroup**.co.in
E-mail & Skype-id: **drkamalkvgroup**@gmail.com
Facebook, WeChat, Youtube, Twitter & Instagram: **drkamalkvgroup**

Acknowledgement

All thanks to almighty (for imparting me with this passion of writing books and teaching), to my parents (for imparting qualities of a good human being), my brothers & sister (for giving me some wonderful memories of childhood), my wife (for supporting me in all my endeavours), my daughters (for allowing me to use their share of time with my students) and my dear students (for accepting my all titles with equal enthusiasm and also, who made me academically strong, to an extent).

Thanks are due for everyone behind this project, from the publication house.

drkamalkv

Contact:
Cell & WhatsApp: 84 7000 4333
Website: www.**drkamalkvgroup**.co.in
E-mail & Skype-id: **drkamalkvgroup**@gmail.com
Facebook, WeChat, Youtube, Twitter & Instagram: **drkamalkvgroup**

Preface

Most of the available titles for FMGE & NEET-PG are MCQs based and many freshers with deficient theoretical concepts found them hard to study. Going after standard textbooks for building concepts is often time consuming and frustrating.

So the need of a concise title focusing on key theoretical topics (related to FMGE & NEET-PG) was felt since long. I have tried to keep the content to a minimum but had tried to put plenty of the stuff which is important from exam (FMGE & NEET-PG) point of view.

For the first edition, I am restricting myself to the most important & commonly asked topics in FMGE & NEET-PG

As I always say, students are the best judge of an authors work. And I personally feel, there is Few more words I always say, "Students are the best judge of an author's work". So please send me your feedbacks/ suggestions/ corrections on my Facebook page "**DRKAMALKVGROUP**".

"To err is human". Despite my best efforts, some errors must have crept in. I request my dear students to please bear with me. Doing a work of such a large volume, makes room for some errors. Please bring them to my knowledge so that I can upload the corrections on my Facebook page. Also I would correct them in subsequent editions.

All the corrections of this title (and my other titles) plus some other exam related information would be updated on my Facebook page "**DRKAMALKVGROUP**" or on my website "**WWW.DRKAMALKVGROUP.CO.IN**". Please follow these and stay updated.

Hope this title serves its purpose.

Once again thanking all my dear students for showering their blessing on me so far & I hope, this sixth edition would also be greeted with the same enthusiasm.

drkamalkv

Classroom Address:

116/3,

Upper Ground floor (Left side),

Near Sribalaji Restaurant,

Sudarshan Road,

Gautam Nagar, New Delhi-49

Remembering our brave soldiers

The **Battle of Longewala** (4–7 December 1971) was one of the first major engagements in the western sector during the Indo-Pakistani War of 1971, fought between assaulting Pakistani forces and Indian defenders at the Indian border post of Longewala, in the Thar Desert of Rajasthan state in India.The battle was fought between 120 Indian soldiers accompanied by 4 Hunter fighter aircraft and 2000-3000 Pakistani soldiers accompanied by 40-45 tanks.

During the night of the 4th, 2Lt. Dharam Veer Bhan's platoon, while on a patrol, detected noises across the border that suggested a large number of armoured vehicles approaching. These were soon confirmed by reports — from the Army's Air Observation Post aircraft flown by Maj. Atma Singh — in the area of a 20 km long armoured column on the track leading to the post advancing in the general direction of the Longewala post. Directing 2Lt. Dharam Veer Bhan's patrol to trail the advancing armoured column, Chandpuri got in touch with battalion headquarters requesting urgent reinforcements and armour and artillery support. Battalion HQ gave him the choice of staying put, and containing the attack as much as possible, or carrying out a tactical retreat of the company to Ramgarh, as reinforcements would not be available for at least six hours. Considering that Chandpuri's command had no transportation, and was facing a mobile enemy, he decided to maintain the defensive position of the post where his troops at least had the benefit of prepared defensive works, rather than conducting a withdrawal at night that was a far riskier option. Chandpuri ensured that all his assets were correctly deployed, and made the most use of his strong defensive position, and weaknesses created by errors in enemy tactics. He was also fortunate in that an Indian Air Force forward air controller was able to secure and direct aircraft in support of the post's defence until reinforcements arrived six hours later.

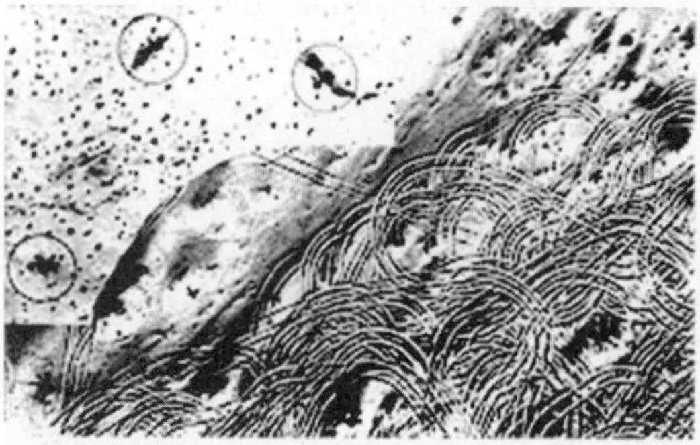

Tank tracks at Longewala. Photographic reconnaissance image taken at the time showing the desperate last minute manoeuvres by Pakistani tanks in the Longewala sector. Circles show destroyed Pakistani tanks

In the morning the Indian Air Force was finally able to direct some HAL HF-24 Maruts and Hawker Hunter aircraft to assist the post; they were not outfitted with night vision equipment, and so were delayed from conducting combat missions until dawn. With daylight, however, the IAF was able to operate effectively, with the strike aircraft being guided to the targets by the airborne Forward Air Controller (FAC) Maj. Atma Singh in a HAL Krishak. The Indian aircraft attacked the Pakistani ground troops with the 16 Matra T-10 rockets and 30 mm cannon fire on each aircraft. Without support from the Pakistan Air Force, which was busy elsewhere, the tanks and other armoured vehicles were easy targets for the IAF's Hunters. The range of the 12.7 mm anti-aircraft heavy machine guns mounted on the tanks was limited and therefore ineffective against the Indian jets. Indian air attacks were made easier by the nature of the barren terrain. Many IAF officers later described the attack as a 'turkey shoot' signifying the lopsidedness. By noon the next day, the assault ended completely, having cost Pakistan 22 tanks claimed destroyed by aircraft fire, 12 by ground anti-tank fire, and some captured after being abandoned, with a total of 100 vehicles claimed to have been destroyed or damaged in the desert around the post. The Pakistani attack was first halted, and then Pakistani forces were forced to withdraw when Indian tanks from the division's cavalry regiment, the 20th Lancers, commanded by Col. Bawa Guruvachan Singh, along with the 17th battalion, Rajputana Rifles, launched their counter-offensive to end the six-hour engagement.

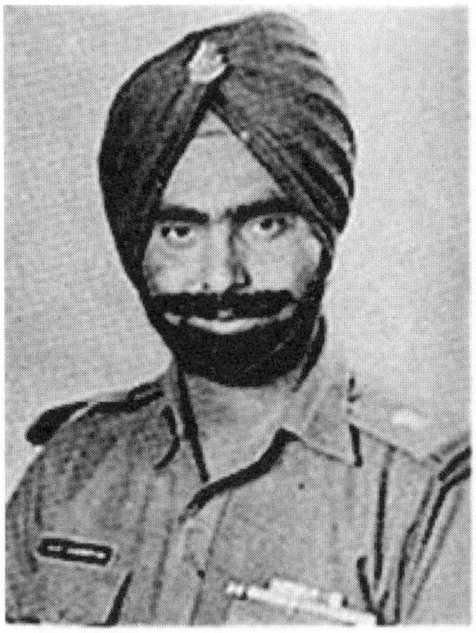
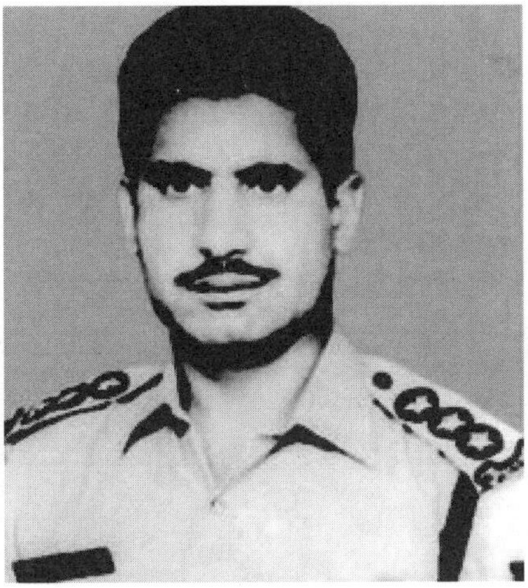
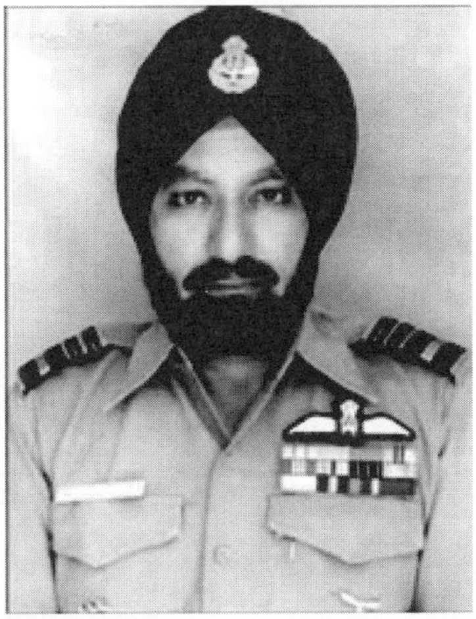

The Battle of Longewala was depicted in the 1997 Bollywood film ***BORDER***, which was directed by J.P. Dutta and starred Sunny Deol as Maj. Kuldip Singh Chandpuri (photo 1), Jackie Shroff as Wg. Cdr. M.S. Bawa (photo 3), Sunil Shetty as Capt. Bhairon Singh (BSF), and the then Akshaye Khanna as Second Lt. Dharam Veer Bhan (photo 2). The main criticism of the movie was that it showed Indian forces being in a terrible position before any sort of help came from the Indian Air Force. The movie also exaggerates the casualties of Indian soldiers for dramatic purposes. This was not the case in the real incident as Indian forces had defended a position on a height that commanded the area, and were able to defend it effectively due to tactical mistakes made by the Pakistani commanders. This resulted in only two sepoys being killed before combat ceased. Indian troops were later able to capture damaged or abandoned Pakistani tanks

I have been to **TANOT KI MATA** temple in Jaisalmer (Rajasthan), which was also depicted in the movie and was lucky to see those bombs which failed to blast (as shown in movie too).

I am a son of ex-armymen & I feel it's my duty to highlight the supreme sacrifices made by our brave soldiers. One can make donations to Indian Army by visiting the website **www.indianarmy.nic.in**

Contents

1.	Anatomy	1
2.	Physiology	20
3.	Biochemistry	34
4.	Pathology	43
5.	Pharmacology	52
6.	Microbiology & Parasitology	67
7.	Forensic Medicine	80
8.	PSM	90

Contents

1.	Anatomy	1
2.	Physiology	20
3.	Biochemistry	34
4.	Pathology	43
5.	Pharmacology	52
6.	Microbiology & Parasitology	67
7.	Forensic Medicine	80
8.	PSM	90

fire, 12 by ground anti-tank fire, and some captured after being abandoned, with a total of 100 vehicles claimed to have been destroyed or damaged in the desert around the post. The Pakistani attack was first halted, and then Pakistani forces were forced to withdraw when Indian tanks from the division's cavalry regiment, the 20th Lancers, commanded by Col. Bawa Guruvachan Singh, along with the 17th battalion, Rajputana Rifles, launched their counter-offensive to end the six-hour engagement.

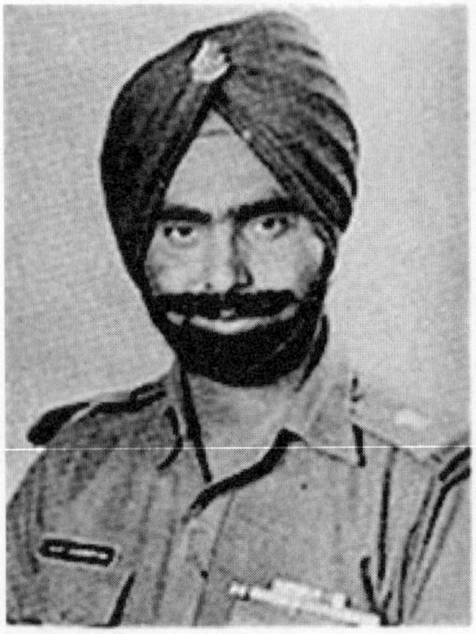
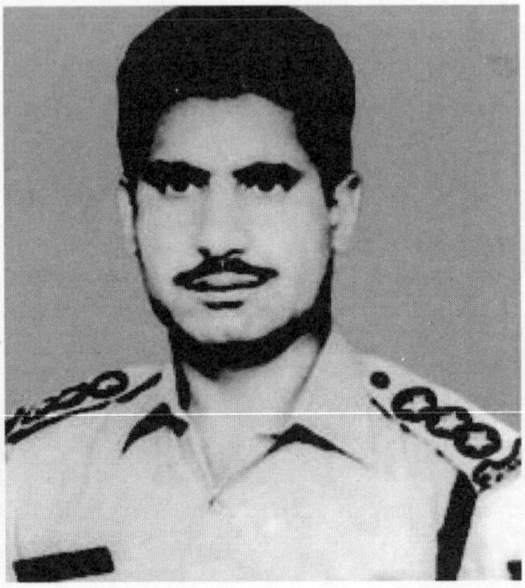
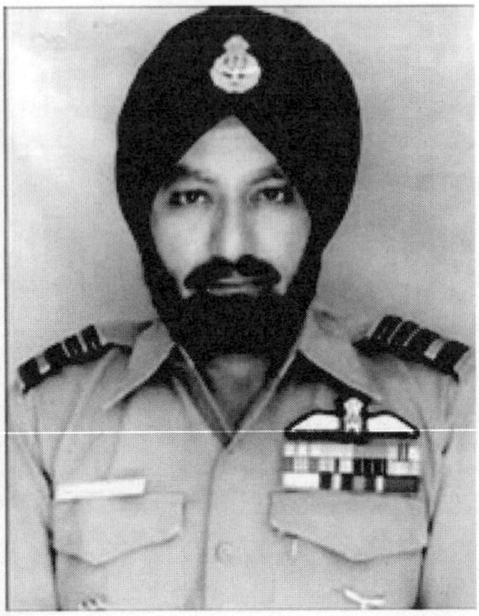

The Battle of Longewala was depicted in the 1997 Bollywood film ***BORDER***, which was directed by J.P. Dutta and starred Sunny Deol as Maj. Kuldip Singh Chandpuri (photo 1), Jackie Shroff as Wg. Cdr. M.S. Bawa (photo 3), Sunil Shetty as Capt. Bhairon Singh (BSF), and the then Akshaye Khanna as Second Lt. Dharam Veer Bhan (photo 2). The main criticism of the movie was that it showed Indian forces being in a terrible position before any sort of help came from the Indian Air Force. The movie also exaggerates the casualties of Indian soldiers for dramatic purposes. This was not the case in the real incident as Indian forces had defended a position on a height that commanded the area, and were able to defend it effectively due to tactical mistakes made by the Pakistani commanders. This resulted in only two sepoys being killed before combat ceased. Indian troops were later able to capture damaged or abandoned Pakistani tanks

I have been to **TANOT KI MATA** temple in Jaisalmer (Rajasthan), which was also depicted in the movie and was lucky to see those bombs which failed to blast (as shown in movie too).

I am a son of ex-armymen & I feel it's my duty to highlight the supreme sacrifices made by our brave soldiers. One can make donations to Indian Army by visiting the website **www.indianarmy.nic.in**

CHAPTER 1

ANATOMY

I. GENERAL ANATOMY

BONE

Parts of a long bone:

- Diaphysis
- Metaphysis
- Epiphysis

Diaphysis:

- Strongest portion
- Contains Haversian canals
- Also known as shaft

Metaphysis:

- Region of active growth
- Highly vascular area
- Lies between epiphysis and diaphysis

Epiphysis:

- Forms the articular end of a long bone
- Covered by articular cartilage

Epiphyseal growth plate:

- Area of longitudinal bone growth
- Present in children only (not in adults)
- Lies between epiphysis and metaphysis

CARTILAGE

Elastic cartilage:

- Present in ear

Fibrocartilage:

- Knee meniscus
- Intervertebral disc
- Glenoidal and acetabular labrum
- Articular disc

Hyaline cartilage:

- Present on articular surfaces of synovial joints
- Respiratory cartilage (trachea, bronchus, larynx, nasal septum)

II. THORAX

SKELETAL FRAMEWORK OF THORAX

True ribs:

- Articulates directly with sternum through costal cartilages
- 1st to 7th ribs are true ribs

False ribs:

- These ribs do not articulate directly with sternum
- 8th to 12th ribs are false ribs

Floating ribs:

- Anterior ends are free
- 11th & 12th

Thoracic vertebrae:

- 12 in number
- Also written as dorsal vertebra
- Contains articular facet for ribs on vertebral bodies

Muscles of thoracic wall:

- External intercostals
- Internal intercostals/ IIC
- Transverse thoracis/ TC
- All muscles are supplied by intercostal nerves
- Neurovascular bundle lies between IIC & TT muscles

VEINS OF THORAX

Azygos vein:

- Begins in abdomen
- Ends by draining into superior vena cava at the level of thoracic vertebra 4/ T4
- Drains blood from the posterior wall of the thorax and abdomen
- Crosses to thorax through aortic hiatus of diaphragm

DIAPHRAGMATIC OPENING

Vena caval opening:

- At the level of T8
- Present in central tendon
- Transmits
  - o Inferior vena cava
  - o Right phrenic nerve

Esophageal hiatus:

- At the level of T10
- Present in muscular portion of diaphragm
- It transmits
  - o Esophagus,
  - o Anterior and posterior vagal trunks

Aortic hiatus:

- Present at the level of T12
- Through osseo-aponeurotic defect (NOT a true opening)
- Transmits
  - o Aorta,
  - o Thoracic duct,
  - o Azygos vein

HEART

Borders:

- Superior border: Formed by right and left atria and auricles in an anterior view
- Inferior border: Formed mainly by the right ventricle and slightly by the left ventricle
- Left border: Formed by the left ventricle and slightly by the left auricle
- Right border: Formed by the right atrium, superior vena cava and inferior vena cava.

Surfaces:

- Base: Formed by left atrium & right atrium
- Apex: Formed by left ventricle
- Inferior surface of the heart is formed by: Both ventricles

Arterial supply of heart:

- Right Coronary artery (Main branches are Posterior Descending & Marginal artery) supplies:
  - o Right atrium & ventricle
  - o Posterior 1/3rd of interventricular septum
  - o SA node (in 60% cases) & AV node
- Left Coronary artery (Main branches are Left Anterior Descending & Circumflex artery) supplies:
  - o Anterior 2/3rd of interventricular septum
  - o SA node (in 40% cases)
  - o Anterior part of right & left ventricle
  - o Lateral wall of left ventricle

Venous drainage of heart:

- 10% drains into heart chambers through venae cordis minimis
- 90% drains through Coronary Sinus into right atrium via Great, Small & Middle cardiac veins (GSM)

THORACIC DUCT

Thoracic duct:

- Thoracic duct crosses from right to left at the level of: T4/ T5

- Thoracic duct passes through which opening: Aortic opening of diaphragm
- Thoracic duct is also known as: Pecquets duct

LUNGS

Right lung:

- Weight: 600 gm
- Has 2 fissures: Horizontal and oblique
- Has 3 lobes: Superior, middle and inferior

Left lung:

- Weight: 565 gm
- Only one fissure (oblique)
- Has 2 lobes: Superior and inferior (an additional lingular lobe)
- Contains cardiac notch

Bronchopulmonary segments:

- Anatomic, functional and surgical unit of the lung
- As it is separated from rest of the lungs by a connective tissue septum, it can be separated surgically without affecting other segments
- It has a segmental bronchus, a segmental artery, lymph vessels and autonomic nerves.
- There are 10 segments on each side

ESOPHAGUS

Anatomy:

- Esophagus pierces diaphragm at a distance of: 15 inches (from incisor)
- Length of esophagus: 25 cm
- Esophagus commences at: Lower end of cricoids
- Epithelium of esophagus: Stratified squamous non-keratinized

Constrictions of esophagus:

- 15 cm (Cricopharynx);
- 25 cm (Aortic arch);
- 27 cm (Left bronchus);
- 40 cm (Diaphragmatic entry)

Esophagus shown three indentations on radiographic study; from above downwards they are:

- Aortic arch;
- Left bronchus;
- Left atrium

Blood supply of esophagus:

- Upper third: Inferior thyroid artery;
- Middle third: Branches from descending thoracic aorta;
- Lower third:Left gastric artery

III. LOWER LIMB

BONES OF LOWER LIMB

Hip bone:

- Ilium
- Ischium
- Pubis

Femur:

- Longest and strongest bone of the body
- In 9th month of intrauterine life, secondary ossification centre appears in lower end
- If fractured, can lead to massive blood loss (around 1.5 L)

Tibia & fibula:

- Bones of leg
- Tibia is medial and fibula is lateral
- Common peroneal nerve winds round the neck of fibula, so all fibular neck fractures should be evaluated for common peroneal nerve injury (foot drop)

Tarsal bones:

- Talus (no muscle attachments)
- Calcaneum (largest)
- Navicular
- Cuboid
- 3 cuneiforms

Metatarsal:

- 5 in number
- Counted from lateral to medial

Phalages:

- 2 in great toe
- 3 in rest of the toes

THIGH

Compartments of thigh & nerve supply:

- Medial/ adductor compartment: Obturator nerve
- Anterior/ Flexor compartment: Femoral nerve
- Posterior/ Hamstrings: Sciatic nerve (Tibial part)

Muscles of the front of thigh:

- Sartorius
- Quadriceps femoris (supplied by femoral nerve)

Quadriceps femoris:

- Rectus femoris
- Vastus medialis
- Vastus intermedius
- Vastus lateralis

Sartorius:

- Origin: ASIS (Anterior superior iliac spine)
- Insertion: Upper part of medial surface of tibia
- Innervated by: Femoral nerve

Hamstring muscles:

- All take origin from ischial tuberosity
- Crosses hip and knee joint and inserts onto tibia/ fibula
- Extends hip and flexes knee
- Innervated by tibial part of the sciatic nerve
- Includes:
  - o Ischial head of adductor magnus
  - o Long head of biceps femoris
  - o Semimembranosus
  - o Semitendinosus

GLUTEAL REGION

Gluteal muscles:

- Gluteus maximus is supplied by: Inferior gluteal nerve
- Gluteus minimus, G. medius & tensor fascia lata is supplied by: Superior gluteal nerve
- Action of gluteus maximus: Extensor of hip joint
- Action of gluteus medius & minimus: Abductor of hip joint

Hip joint:

- Superior & inferior gemelli and piriformis action: Lateral rotation
- Abductors of the hip: Gluteus medius & gluteus minimus
- Function of ileofemoral ligament/ ligament of Bigelow (strongest ligament in the body): Prevents hyperextension at the hip (prevents backward falling of trunk)

KNEE

Knee joint:

- Extensor of the knee joint: Quadricep femoris
- Posterior dislocation of femur is prevented by: Anterior cruciate ligament
- Posterior dislocation of the tibia is prevented by: Posterior cruciate ligament
- Medial meniscus tears are more common than lateral meniscus because medial meniscus is attached to tibial collateral ligament
- Locking of knee: Vastus medialis
- Unlocking of knee: Popliteus

Bursitis around knee joint:

- Subcutaneous infrapatellar bursa: Clergyman's knee
- Subcutaneous prepatellar bursa: Housemaid's knee

FOOT

Joints of the foot:

- Dorsiflexion & plantarflexion of foot occurs at: Ankle joint
- Inversion & eversion occurs at: Subtalar joint and midtarsal (talo-calcaneo-navicular and calcaneo-cuboid) joints
- Inversion is produced by:
  - o Tibialis anterior &
  - o tibialis posterior
- Eversion is produced by: Peronei (P. longus, P. brevis and P. tertius)

NERVES OF LOWER LIMB

Obturator nerve:

- Supplies muscle of medial compartment of thigh
- It has 2 divisions:
  - o Anterior
  - o Posterior
- Adductor magnus is also supplied by posterior division of obturator nerve
- Sometimes TB hip (other pathologies) may cause referred pain in the knee joint because obturator nerve supplies both joints.

LEG

Fascial compartments of leg & Innervation of muscles:

- Anterior compartment: Deep peroneal nerve
- Lateral compartment: Superficial peroneal nerve
- Posterior compartment: Tibial nerve

FEMORAL TRIANGLE

Boundaries:

- Inguinal ligament forms the upper border
- Sartorius forms the lateral border
- Medial border of adductor longus forms the medial border

Contents:

- Femoral nerve, artery and vein
- Femoral sheath
- Femoral canal
- Deep inguinal nodes

ADDUCTOR CANAL

Contents:

- Terminal part of femoral artery
- Femoral vein
- Saphenous nerve
- Nerve to vastus medialis
- Terminal part of obturator nerve
- Deep lymph vessels

TRENDELENBERG TEST

Trendelenberg test:

- If a subject stands on one leg, pelvis on the opposite side tends to sag because of gravity.
- But the abductor muscles (gluteus medius and minimus) of the same side (on which the patient is standing) pulls the pelvis and counteract this tendency of sagging down.
- If the abductor mechanism is defective (paralysis of muscles, fracture neck of femur or congenital dislocation of hip), opposite side pelvis sags down and this is known as positive Trendelenburg test.
- Landmark noted is anterior superior iliac spine/ ASIS.
- This test should not be confused with Brodie-Trendelenberg test which checks sapheno-femoral competence.

IV. ABDOMEN & PELVIS

ABDOMINAL QUADRANTS

Planes of abdomen:

- Two vertical midclavicular planes
- Two horizontal planes:

- o Upper subcostal and
- o Lower transtubercular plane

9 Quadrants:

- Epigastrium
- Right & left hypochondrium
- Umbilical
- Right& left lumbar
- Hypogastrium
- Right & left iliac fossa

ANTERIOR ABDOMINAL WALL

Superficial fascia is divided into:

- Camper's fascia:
- Superficial fatty layer

Muscles of anterior abdomen:

- External oblique
- Internal oblique
- Transversus abdominis
- Rectus abdominis (6-pack)
- Pyramidalis

POSTERIOR ABDOMINAL WALL

Contains:

- Lumbar vertebrae
- Intervertebral disc
- Muscles:
  - o Psoas major,
  - o Quadratus lumborum,
  - o Iliacus etc.

STOMACH

Blood supply of the stomach:

- Right gastric artery (Hepatic artery) supplies: Lower right part of the stomach
- Short gastric artery (Splenic artery) supplies: Fundus
- Left gastric artery (Celiac artery) supplies: Lower third of esophagus upper right part of the stomach
- Left gastroepiploic artery (Splenic artery) supplies: Upper part of greater curvature
- Right gastroepiploic artery (Gastroduodenal artery) supplies: Lower part of greater curvature

DUODENUM/ D

Divided into four parts:

- D1 (superior part): 5 cm
- D2 (descending part): 7.5 cm
- D3 (horizontal part): 10 cm
- D4 (ascending part): 2.5 cm

Brunners gland:

- Main function of these glands is to produce mucus rich alkaline secretion which protects duodenum from gastric acid.

RECTUM

Parts of rectum:

- Upper one-third is covered by peritoneum on anterior surface
- Middle third is covered by peritoneum on anterior surface
- Lower third is not covered by peritoneum hence it is the most mobile part

LIVER

Anatomy:

- Liver is divided into right and left lobes by the attachment of the peritoneum of the falciform ligament.
- The right lobe is further divided into a quadrate lobe and caudate lobe, by gallbladder, fissure for the ligamentum teres, the inferior vena cava and the fissure for ligamentum venosum.

CALOT'S TRIANGLE/ CYSTOHEPATIC TRIANGLE/ HEPATOBILIARY TRIANGLE

Bounded by:

- Inferior surface of liver superiorly
- Cystic duct inferolaterally
- Common hepatic duct medially

Content:

- Cystic artery
- Lymph node of Lund
- Right hepatic artery

KIDNEY

Coverings of kidney from inside outside are:

- Fibrous capsule
- Perirenal fat
- Renal fascia (fascia of Gerota)
- Pararenal fat (Fascia of Zuckerlandl is the posterior layer of ranal fascia)

The renal hilum transmits following structures from front to backwards:

- Renal vein
- Two branches of the renal artery
- Ureter
- Third branch of the renal artery

Tributaries of left renal vein:

- Left gonadal vein
- Left suprarenal vein
- Left inferior phrenic vein

Renal transplantation:

- Left kidney is selected for transplantation
- Iliac fossa is the preferred site for transplanted kidney

URETER

3 constrictions:

- Where the renal pelvis joins the ureter;
- Where it crosses the pelvic brim;
- Where it enters the urinary bladder wall

ADRENAL GLAND

Arterial supply:

- Branch of Phrenic artery supplies superior part
- Direct branch from aorta supplies middle part
- Branch of renal artery supplies lower part

Venous drainage:

- Left suprarenal gland drains into left renal vein
- Right suprarenal gland drains into inferior vena cava.

SPERMATIC CORD

Constituents of spermatic cord:

- Ductus deferens
- Testicular and cremasteric arteries and artery of the ducts deferens
- Pampiniform plexus of veins
- Lymph vessels from testis
- Plexus of sympathetic nerves around the artery to the ductus deferens
- Remains of processus vaginalis

Coverings of the spermatic cord:

- External spermatic fascia: Derived from external oblique aponeurosis
- Cremasteric fascia: Derived from internal oblique aponeurosis
- Internal spermatic fascia: Derived from fascia transversalis

ARTERIES OF ABDOMEN

Branches of Coeliac trunk:

- Splenic artery
- Left gastric artery
- Common hepatic artery

Branches of splenic artery:

- Left gastro-epiploic artery
- Short gastric branches
- Pancreatic branches

Branches of common hepatic artery:

- Gastroduodenal artery
- Right & left hepatic artery
- Cystic artery
- Right gastric artery

PELVIS & PERINEUM

Uterus:

- Size: 3 × 2 × 1 inch
- Weight: 30 – 40 gm
- Position: 90 degree forward with long axis of vagina

Cervix:

- Size: 2.5 cm
- Lining:
  - o Ectocervix: Non-keratinized stratified squamous
  - o Endocervix: Simple columnar

MALE URETHRA

4 parts:

- Penile
- Bulbar
- Membranous (least dilatable)
- Prostatic (most wide)

PROSTATE

Lobes of prostate:

- Anterior lobe;
- Median / middle lobe (enlarged in BPH);
- Posterior lobe (most common site of malignancy);
- Right and left lateral lobes

UROGENITAL DIAPHRAGM

Formed by:

- Superior fascia of urogenital diaphragm
- Perineal membrane
- Sphincter urethrae
- Deep transverse perineii

PERINEAL BODY

Formed by:

- External anal sphincter
- Sphincter urethrae
- Deep transverse perineii
- Superficial transverse perineii
- Bulbospongiosus
- Levator ani muscle (ilio-coccygeus & pubo-coccygeus)

V. HEAD & NECK

SKULL BONES

Divided into:

- Cerebral cranium
- Facial cranium

Paired bones of cerebral cranium:

- Parietal
- Temporal

Unpaired bones of cerebral cranium:

- Occipital
- Sphenoid
- Ethmoid
- Frontal

Paired bones of facial cranium:

- Maxilla
- Lacrimal
- Zygomatic
- Palatine
- Nasal
- Inferior nasal concha

Unpaired bones of facial cranium:

- Hyoid
- Mandible
- Vomer

TEMPORO-MANDIBULAR JOINT

Movements & muscles:

- Depressor: Lateral pterygoid
- Protrusion: Pterygoids (Medial & lateral)
- Retraction: Posterior fibres of temporalis

SCALP

Layers of SCALP:

- S: Skin (contains hair follicles)
- C: Connective tissue (highly vascular)
- A: Aponeurosis/ Gala aponeurotica
- L: Loose areolar tissue (dangerous area of scalp)
- P: Pericranium (periosteum of skull bones)

SKULL FORMINA

Skull foramina & structures passing through them:

- Carotid canal: Internal carotid artery
- Foramen rotundum: Maxillary nerve
- Foramen lacerum:
  - o Internal carotid artery,
  - o Nerve of pterygoid canal
- Jugular foramen:
  - o Inferior petrosal sinus,
  - o 9th, 10th, 11th cranial nerves,
  - o Internal jugular vein
- Stylomastoid foramen: Facial nerve
- Foramen magnum:
  - o Medulla,
  - o Tonsils of cerebellum,
  - o Meninges.
- Through subarachnoid space in foramen magnum:
  - o Spinal accessory nerve,
  - o Vertebral artery,
  - o Posterior spinal artery
  - o Anterior spinal artery.
- Through anterior part of foramen magnum:
  - o Ligament of dens,
  - o Membrana tectoria.
- Optic canal: Optic nerve
- Superior orbital fissure:
  - o Superior ophthalmic vein,
  - o Lacrimal nerve,
  - o Frontal nerve,
  - o Trochlear nerve,
  - o Oculomotor nerve,
  - o Nasociliary nerve,
  - o Abducent nerves
- Hypoglossal canal: Hypoglossal nerve
- Internal acoustic meatus: Vestibulocochlear and facial nerve
- Foramen spinosum:
  - o Middle meningial artery,
  - o Nervous spinosus and
  - o Posterior trunk of middle meningeal artery
- Foramen ovale:
  - o Mandibular nerve,
  - o Accessory meningeal artery,
  - o Lesser petrosal nerve,
  - o Vein connecting cavernous sinus with the pterygoid plexus of veins

EXTERNAL CAROTID ARTERY

Branches of external carotid artery:

- Anterior:
  - o Superior thyroid artery,
  - o Lingual artery,
  - o Facial artery
- Posterior:
  - o Occipital artery,
  - o Posterior auricular artery
- Medial:
  - o Ascending pharyngeal
- Terminal:
  - o Maxillary artery,
  - o Superficial temporal artery

TONGUE

Sensory innervation of tongue:

- Anterior 2/ 3rd (including circumvallate papillae for taste sensation):
  - o Lingual nerve for general sensation;
  - o Chorda tympani branch of facial nerve for taste sensation
- Posterior 1/ 3rd (except circumvallate papillae for taste sensation): Glosso-pharyngeal nerve for both general sensation & taste sensation

EYE

Movements of eyeball & muscles:

- Extorters of eyeball: Both Inferior's
- Intorters of eye: Both Superior's

Actions of extraocular muscles:

- Superior rectus: Moves eyeball upward and medially
- Inferior rectus: Moves eyeball downwards and medially
- Medial rectus: Moves eyeball medially
- Lateral rectus: Moves eyeball laterally
- Inferior oblique: Moves eyeball upwards and laterally
- Superior oblique:
  - o Abduction,
  - o Intorsion &
  - o Depression

Other muscles related to eyeball:

- Muller's muscle:
  - o Attached to posterior tarsal margin
  - o Supplied by sympathetic plexus
- Orbicularis oculi:
  - o Supplied by Facial nerve;
  - o Closes eyeball and dilates lacrimal sac
- Levator Palpebrae Superioris:
  - o Supplied by oculomotor nerve;
  - o Raises upper lid and sympathetic supply
- Sphincter Pupillae:
  - o Parasympathetic supply;
  - o Constricts pupil by oculomotor nerve
- Dilator pupillae:
  - o Sympathetic supply;
  - o Dilates pupil
- Ciliary muscle:
  - o Parasympathetic supply by occulomotor nerve;
  - o Controls shape of eye,
  - o Helps in accommodation

Nerve supply of extraocular muscles:

- SO-4 (superior oblique by trochlear nerve)
- LR-6 (lateral rectus by abducens nerve)
- Rest by 3 (rest of the muscles by oculomotor nerve)

SALIVARY GLANDS

Parotid gland:

- Duct: Stenson's duct
- Opening of duct: Vestibule of mouth, opposite the crown of upper second molar tooth

Submandibular gland:

- Duct: Wharton's duct
- Opening of duct: Floor of mouth, on the summit of the sublingual papilla at the side of frenulum (tongue)

NECK

Movements of neck:

- Rotational movement (saying NO/ dis-approval): Atlanto-axial joint
- Flexion & extension (saying YES/ approval/ nodding): Atlanto-occipital joint

LARYNX

Sensory innervations:

- Above the level of vocal cords is by: Internal laryngeal nerve
- Below the level of vocal cords: Recurrent laryngeal nerve

Muscles of larynx:

- Nerve supply of cricothyroid: External laryngeal nerve
- Abductor of vocal cords: Posterior crico-arytenoid
- Adductor of vocal cords:
  - o Lateral crico-arytenoids
  - o Transverse arytenoids
- Tensor of vocal cords: Crico-thyroid

TRACHEA

Anatomy:

- Begins at: Lower border of cricoids cartilage (C6 vertebrae)

- Extent of trachea: C6 to T5
- Bifurcation of trachea: T4/ T5
- Length of trachea: 10-12 cm
- Trachea has C shaped tracheal rings, which are posteriorly completed into a ring by trachealis muscle.

THYROID GLAND

Anatomy:

- Located in anterior triangle of the neck
- Weight: 20 grams
- Extent: C5 to T1 vertebrae
- Two lobes are connected by isthmus
- Isthmus extends from 2nd to 4th tracheal rings

Blood supply of thyroid gland:

- Superior thyroid artery (branch of external carotid artery)
- Inferior thyroid artery (branch of thyrocervical trunk of subclavian artery)
- Thyroidea ima artery (branch of aorta/ brachiocephalic artery)

Cells of thyroid:

- Parafollicular/ C cells secrete: Calcitonin
- Follicular cells secrete: T3 and T4.

CAROTID SHEATH

Contents of carotid sheath:

- Carotid arteries (within the sheath common carotid divides into external and internal carotids)
- Internal jugular vein
- Vagus nerve

VI. BRAIN & SPINAL CORD

CEREBRAL HEMISPHERES

Nuclei:

- Nucleus dentatus
- Nucleus emboliformis
- Nucleus globosus
- Nucleus fastigii

TRIGEMINAL NERVE

Branches & openings through which they pass:

- Mandibular: Foramen ovale
- Maxillary: Foramen rotundum
- Ophthalmic: Superior orbital fissure

CRANIAL NERVES

Cranial nerves & their nuclei:

- Nerves having nuclei in midbrain: III, IV
- Nerves having nuclei in pons: V, VI, VII, VIII
- Nerves having nuclei in medulla: IX, X, XI, XII

MENINGES

3 layers:

- Innermost Piamater
- Arachnoid mater
- Outer duramater
- Middle arachnoid & inner piamater together are known as leptomeninges

INTERNAL CAPSULE

Genu of internal capsule contains fibres of:

- Descending tracts: Corticonulcear fibres (Supranuclear pathway)
- Ascending tracts: Sensory fibres/ Anterior part of superior thalamic radiation (from thalamus to brain)

Other parts of internal capsule:

- Retro-lentiform part of internal capsule contains: Optic radiation
- Sub-lentiform part of internal capsule contains: Auditory radiation

ARTERIES OF BRAIN

Effect of blockage of arteries:

- Left middle cerebral artery blockage results in: Right sided hemiplegia, sensory deficits (face & arm)
- Right middle cerebral artery blockage results in: Left side hemiplegia, sensory deficits (face & arm)
- Right posterior cerebral artery blockade results in: Left sided visual field defect
- Medial medullary syndrome is due to occlusion of: Vertebral artery
- Lateral medullary syndrome is due to occlusion of: Posterior inferior cerebellar artery

CRANIAL NERVES

Olfactory:

- Sensory
- Perceives smell

Optic:

- Sensory
- Vision

Oculomotor:

- Motor
- Supplies levator palpebrae superioris, superior rectus, medial rectus, inferior rectus, inferior oblique,
- Supplies sphincter pupillae and ciliary muscle with parasymapathetic fibres

Trochlear:

- Motor
- Supplies superior oblique

Trigeminal:

- Mixed
- Supplies sensory fibres to the skin of the scalp, face, mouth, teeth, nasal cavity and paranasal sinuses; supplies motor fibres to the muscles of mastication, tensor veli palatini and tensor tympani

Abducent:

- Motor
- Supplies lateral rectus

Facial:

- Mixed
- Supplies motor fibres to the muscles of face, scalp with auricle, buccinator, platysma, stapedius, stylohyoid and posterior belly of digastric;
- Gives sensory supply to anterior 2/3rd of tongue, floor of mouth and the palate;
- Gives parasympathetic secretomotor fibres to the submandibular and sublingual salivary glands, lacrimal glands and the glands of the nose and palate

Vestibulocochlear:

- Sensory
- Position and movement of head
- Hearing

Glossopharyngeal:

- Mixed
- Supplies stylopharyngeus muscle
- Supplies parasympathetic secretomotor fibres to the parotid gland, sensory and taste fibres to the posterior third of tongue and pharynx.

Vagus:

- Mixed
- Supplies constrictor muscles of pharynx and intrinsic muscles of larynx
- Supplies involuntary muscles of trachea and bronchi, heart, alimentary tract from pharynx to splenic flexure of colon, liver and pancreas;
- Afferent fibres from the abdominal structures,
- Taste fibres from epiglottis and velleculae

Spinal accessory:

- Motor
- Supplies sternocleidomastoid and trapezius.

Hypoglossal:

- Motor
- Supplies muscles of tongue except palato-glossus.

CEREBROSPINAL FLUID

CSF:

- It is principally secreted by: Choroid plexus
- Choroid plexus is absent in: Anterior horn of lateral ventricle
- Total volume of CSF: 150 ml
- pH of CSF: 7.33
- Main factor controlling CSF pressure: Rate of CSF absorption
- Neurtophils in CSF: Are normally absent

BRAIN

Brodman areas:

- Primary auditory area is in (41, 42, 22): Superior part of the temporal gyrus
- Primary visual area is in (17): Occipital lobe
- Broacas area is in (44, 45): Inferior frontal gyrus
- Loss of tactile localization & 2 point discrimination occurs in damage to: Somatosensory area 1

VISUAL PATHWAY

Lesion of visual pathway:

- Optic nerve: Blindness in that eye
- Crossing fibres of optic chiasma: Bitemporal hemianopia
- Lateral parts of chiasma: Binasal hemianopia
- Optic tract/ lateral geniculate body: Contralateral homonymous hemianopia
- Meyer's loop of optic radiation: Contralateral superior quadrantic anopia
- Vascular lesion of occipital lobe: Contralateral homonymous hemianopia with macula sparing

BLOOD BRAIN BARRIER

Blood-brain barrier is absent at:

- Pituitary
- Area postrema
- Organuma vasculosum of lamina terminalis
- Subfornical organ
- Ventral part of median eminence of hypothalamus
- Anterior pituitary
- Pineal gland

SPINAL CORD

Level of spinal cord termination:

- In adults: Terminates at the lower end of L1
- In children: Terminates at the lower end of L3

Arterial supply of spinal cord:

- Three major longitudinal vessels (originating from vertebral artery):
  - o Single anterior spinal artery
  - o Two posterior spinal arteries

VII. UPPER LIMB

BONES OF UPPER EXTREMITY

Pectoral girdle:

- Clavicle and
- Scapula

Upper limb includes:

- Arm (humerus),
- Forearm (radius and ulna) and
- Hand (carpals, metacarpals and phalanges)

CLAVICLE

Peculiarities of clavicle:

- Transmits weight of upper limb to axial skeleton through coraco-clavicular ligament

- Only long bone to lie horizontally
- No medullary cavity
- Membranous ossification
- First bone to ossify
- Fractures commonly at junction of medial 2/3rd and lateral 1/3rd
- Most common bone to fracture in body

SCAPULA

Muscle originating from coracoid process:

- Origin:
  - o Short head of biceps,
  - o Coracobrachialis
- Insertion:
  - o Pectoralis minor

Ligaments attached to coracoid process:

- Coraco-clavicular ligament: Transmits weight of upper limb to clavicle
- Coraco-acromial ligament: Prevents superior displacement of humeral head

Vertebral levels & landmarks of scapula:

- D7: Inferior angle
- D3: Root of spinous process
- T2: Superior angle

HUMERUS

Attachments of humerus:

- Muscles attached to greater tubercle of humerus:
  - o Supraspinatus,
  - o Infraspinatus &
  - o Teres minor
- Structures attached on intertubercular sulcus:
  - o Lateral lip: Pectoralis major
  - o Floor: Latissimus dorsi
  - o Medial lip: Teres major
- Structures attached on lesser tubercle: Subscapularis

Structures related to humerus:

- Structures related to surgical neck of humerus:
  - o Anterior and posterior circumflex vessels
  - o Axillary nerve
- Structures lying in radial groove:
  - o Profunda brachii vessels
  - o Radial nerve

Nerves related to humerus:

- Posterior aspect of surgical neck: Axillary nerve
- Radial/ spiral groove: Radial nerve
- Posterior aspect of medial epicondyle: Ulnar nerve

CARPALS

Lateral to medial:

- Proximal row: Scaphoid, lunate, triquetral, pisiform
- Distal row: Trapezium, trapezoid, capitate, hamate

Carpal bones:

- Largest carpal bone: Capitate
- Most common carpal bone to dislocate: Lunate
- Most common carpal bone to fracture: Scaphoid

BRACHIAL PLEXUS

Parts:

- RTDC (Roots, Trunks, Division, Cords)

Location:

- Roots and trunks in neck
- Divisions behind the clavicle
- Cords in axilla

Injuries:

- Upper trunk injury: Policeman's tip hand
- Lower trunk injury: Klumpke's palsy
- Long thoracic nerve injury: Winging of scapula

Deformities following nerve injuries:

- Ape hand: Median nerve injury
- Partial clawing: Ulnar nerve injury
- Complete clawing: Both ulnar & median nerve injury
- Wrist drop: Radial nerve injury

Erb's palsy:

- Involves upper trunk of brachial plexus
- Nerves & Muscles paralyzed:
  - o Suprascapular nerve (Supraspinatus & Infraspinatus)
  - o Axillary nerve (Deltoid & Teres minor)
  - o Musculocutaneous nerve (Biceps brachii, coracobrachialis & brachio-radialis)
  - o Nerve to subclavius (Subclavius muscle)
- Waiters tip deformity/ Policeman or Waiters tip deformity:
  - o Loss of abduction of arm (Deltoid & supraspinatus)
  - o Loss of lateral rotation of arm (Teres minor & infraspinatus)
  - o Loss of flexion of elbow (Biceps brachii, coracobrachialis & brachioradialis)

Klumpke's paralysis:

- Injury to lower trunk of brachial plexus (C8,T1)
- Results in clawing of hand and Horner's syndrome

SHOULDER JOINT

Shoulder joint:

- Type: Synovial ball & socket
- Shoulder joint is weakest: Inferiorly (Shoulder joint is MC dislocated inferiorly due to laxity of capsule and absence of the musculotendinous cuff inferiorly)
- Flexion at shoulder joint is carried out by:
  - o Clavicular head of pectoralis major,
  - o Anterior fibres of deltoid
- Shoulder joint is unstable: As glenoid cavity is shallow
- Most common type of shoulder joint: Antero-inferiorly
- Nerve commonly injured in anterior shoulder dislocation: Axillary nerve
- Luxatio erecta: Inferior dislocation of shoulder joint

Abductors of shoulder joint:

- Initiation (0 – 15 degree): Supraspinatus
- 15-90 degree: Deltoid
- >90 degree:
  - o Serratus anterior
  - o Trapezius

Rotator cuff muscles:

- Tendons of 4 muscles blend with the capsule and form the cuff
- Muscles are
  - o Supraspinatus (superiorly),
  - o Infraspinatus &
  - o Teres minor (posteriorly)
  - o Subscapularis (anteriorly)

JOINTS OF UPPER LIMB

Joints & types:

- Acromio-clavicular joint: Plane synovial joint
- Sterno-clavicular joint: Saddle synovial joint
- Elbow joint: Hinge synovial joint
- Superior/ Proximal & Inferior/ distal radio-ulnar joint: Pivot synovial joint
- Radio-carpal joint: Condyloid synovial joint
- Intercarpal joints & Carpo-metacarpal joints (2nd to 5th): Plane synovial joint
- 1st Carpo-metacarpal joint (Trapezium with 1st metacarpal): Saddle synovial joint
- Metacarpo-phalangeal joints: Condyloid synovial joint
- Inter-phalangeal joint: Hinge synovial joint

MUSCLES OF ARM

Anterior compartment (all supplied by musculocutaneous nerve):

- Brachialis

- Coracobrachialis
- Biceps brachii

Posterior compartment:

- Triceps (supplied by radial nerve)

Flexors of forearm:

- Biceps,
- Brachialis,
- Brachioradialis (3B)

CUBITAL FOSSA

Boundaries:

- Lateral: Brachioradialis
- Superior: Line across epicondyles
- Medial: Pronator teres

Contents:

- Tendon of biceps brachii
- Median nerve
- Brachial artery
- Radial nerve

MUSCLES OF ANTERIOR COMPARTMENT OF FOREARM

Superficial group:

- Palmaris longus
- Pronator teres
- Flexor carpi radialis
- Flexor carpi ulnaris
- Flexor digitorum superficialis

Deep group:

- Flexor digitroum profundus
- Flexor pollicis longus
- Pronator quadratus

MUSCLES OF POSTERIOR COMPARTMENT OF FOREARM

Superficial compartment:

- Brachioradialis
- Anconeus
- Extensor carpi ulnaris
- Extensor digitorum
- Extensor digiti minimi
- Extensor carpi radialis longus
- Extensor carpi radialis brevis

Deep compartment:

- Supinator
- Extensor pollicis longus
- Extensor pollicis brevis
- Extensor indicis
- Abductor pollicis longus

HAND

Dorsal interossei:

- 4 bipennate muscles
- Abduction of fingers

Palmar interossei:

- 3 unipennate muscles
- Adduction of fingers

Ulnar nerve:

- All the intrinsic muscles of the palm are supplied by ulnar nerve except LOFA
- 1st and 2nd lumbricals
- Opponens pollicis
- Flexor pollicis brevis (superficial head)
- Abductor pollicis brevis

Thenar muscles:

- Abductor pollicis and opponens pollicis are supplied by median nerve
- Flexor pollicis brevis:
  - Superficial head is supplied by median nerve
  - Deep head is supplied by ulnar nerve

CARPAL TUNNEL

Structure passing through carpal tunnel:

- Flexor digitorum profundus
- Flexor digitorum superficialis

- Flexor pollicis longus
- Median nerve

ANATOMICAL SNUFF BOX

Boundaries:

- Medial: Extensor pollicis longus
- Lateral: Extensor pollicis brevis
- Floor: Scaphoid, styloid of radius

Contents:

- Cephalic vein
- Radial nerve
- Radial artery

RADIAL NERVE

Muscles Supplied:

- Triceps
- Extensors of metacarpo-phalangeal joint (Extensor compartment of arm & forearm)
- Anconeus

Injury in axillary part:

- Loss of elbow extension
- Wrist drop
- Finger drop
- Loss of cutaneous sensations

Injury in fracture shaft of humerus:

- Wrist drop
- Finger drop
- Loss of cutaneous sensations

Injury in forearm:

- Finger drop
- Loss of cutaneous sensations

Injury at wrist:

- Loss of cutaneous sensations

MEDIAN/ LABOURER'S NERVE

Muscle supplied in forearm:

- All muscles of flexor compartment of forearm except medial half of flexor digitorum profundus

Muscle supplied in hand (LOFA):

- 1st and 2nd lumbrical
- Opponens pollicis
- Flexor pollicis brevis
- Abductor pollicis brevis

Injury results in:

- Ape thumb deformity
- Pointing index
- Loss of opposition and thumb abduction

ULNAR/ MUSICIAN'S NERVE

Muscle supplied in hand:

- All muscles except LOFA
    - o 1st and 2nd lumbrical
    - o Opponens pollicis
    - o Flexor pollicis brevis
    - o Abductor pollicis brevis

Cubital tunnel syndrome:

- Compression neuropathy of ulnar nerve
- Ulnar nerve pierces flexor carpi ulnaris and can be compressed

Injury results in:

- Partial clawing of hand
- Involving 4th & 5th finger

Clinical tests related to ulnar nerve:

- Book test/ Froment sign
- Egawa test
- Card test

VIII. HISTOLOGY

EPITHELIUM

Simple squamous epithelium:

- Endocardium
- Endothelium
- Ansa nephroni

Simple cuboid epithelium:

- Proximal & distal convoluted tubules

- Collecting ducts
- Follicles of thyroid gland

Ciliated simple columnar epithelium:

- Fallopian tube
- Efferent ductile of testis

Simple columnar epithelium with brush border:

- Gall bladder

Stratified squamous, keratinized epithelium:

- Skin
- Duct of sebaceous glands

Stratified squamous, non-keratinized epithelium:

- Tongue
- Esophagus
- Tonsil
- Vagina
- Cornea
- Conjunctiva

Stratified cuboid epithelium:

- Sweat gland
- Pancreas

Stratified columnar epithelium:

- Part of male urethra

Transitional epithelium:

- Renal pelvis till proximal part of urethra (include ureter, urinary bladder)

Pseudocolumnar epithelium:

- Respiratory tract
- Auditory tube
- Vas deferens
- Major portion of urethra in males and females

HISTOLOGICAL FEATURES

Histological features & related structures:

- Intercalated disc is present in: Cardiac muscle
- Nucleus in cardiac muscle: Central
- Reticulo-endothelial cells of liver are: Kupffer cells
- Space of Disse & space of Mall are seen in: Liver
- Intrinsic factor (Castle) is secreted by: Parietal/ oxyntic cells
- Hassal's corpuscles: Thymus
- PALS/ Periarteriolar lymphoid sheath: Spleen
- Brunner's gland: Duodenum
- Peyer's patches: Ileum

IX. EMBRYOLOGY

SPERMATOGENESIS & OOGENESIS

Sperm:

- Stored in: Epididymis
- Acquires motility in: Epididymis
- Capacitation (acquiring capacity to fertilize ovum) occurs in: Fallopian tube
- Length of mature sperm: 50 – 60 microns

Oogenesis:

- First polar body is released at the time of: Ovulation (some says 24 hours prior to ovulation)
- Second polar body is released at the time of: Fertilization
- Oogonia & germ cell are derived from: Yolk sac
- 1st polar body is formed during: Oogenesis

FETAL STRUCTURES & ADULT REMNANTS

Adult remnants & fetal structures:

- Meckel's divertculum: Remnant of vitelline duct
- Ligamentum venosum: Remnant of ductus venosus
- Ligamentum arteriosum: Remnant of ductus arteriosus

- Median umbilical ligament: Remnant of urachus
- Medial umbilical ligaments: Remnant of 2 umbilical arteries

DERIVATIVES OF GERM LAYERS

Structures & germ layers:

- Trigone of bladder: Mesoderm
- Somites: Paraxial mesoderm
- Tympanic membrane: All the 3 germ layers

Derivatives of neural crest:

- Neurons of dorsal root, sensory & autonomic/ sympathetic ganglia,
- Schwann cells,
- Melanocytes,
- Mesenchyme of dental papillae etc.

PHARYNGEAL ARCHES

Structures & derived from (Pharyngeal arch):

- Meckel's cartilage develops from: 1st pharyngeal arch
- Sphenomandibular ligament develops from: 1st pharyngeal arch
- Stapes develops from: 2nd pharyngeal arch
- Stylohyoid ligament develops from: 2nd pharyngeal arch
- Greater cornua of hyoid develops from: 3rd pharyngeal arch
- Posterior belly of digastric develops from: 2nd pharyngeal arch
- Anterior belly of digastric develops from:
- 1st pharyngeal arch
- Platysma develops from: 2nd pharyngeal arch

Nerve supply of derivatives of pharyngeal arches:

- 1st arch: Mandibular nerve
- 2nd arch: Facial nerve
- 3rd arch: Glossopharyngeal nerve
- 6th arch: Recurrent laryngeal nerve

PHARYNGEAL POUCHES

Structures & derivative of (pharyngeal pouch):

- Palatine tonsil develops from: 2nd pharyngeal pouch
- Inferior parathyroid gland & thymus develops from: 3rd pharyngeal pouch
- 4th + 5th pharyngeal pouch forms Caudal pharyngeal complex & forms
  - o Superior parathyroid
  - o Parafollicular cells of thyroid

CHAPTER 2

PHYSIOLOGY

I. GENERAL PHYSIOLOGY

CELLULAR PHYSIOLOGY

3 major class of molecules:

- Structural fibrous proteins (collagen, elastin, fibrillin),
- Adhesive glycoproteins (fibronectin, laminin) &
- Glycans (hyaluronic acid, chondroitin sulfate, heparan sulfate)

Cytoskeletal elements:

- Microtubule (Cilia, flagella, mitotic spindles etc.)
- Actin & myosin (Muscle contraction)

CELL ORAGENELLES & FUNCTIONS

Agranular endoplasmic reticulum:

- Synthesis of lipids (steroid hormones, membrane phospholipid & cholesterols)
- Site of fatty acid elongation, drug detoxification

Rough ER:

- Synthesis of proteins (secretory/ exported, cell membrane) & lysosomal enzymes
- Site of co-transitional modifications of proteins (hydroxylation of proline & lysine during collagen synthesis),
- Initial folding of polypeptide chain proteins into 3D structure

Microtubules:

- Cell shape & motility
- Chediak Higashi syndrome is due to microtubule polymerization defect (impaired phagocytosis)
- Drugs which acts of microtubules: Mebendazole, Colchicine, Thiabendazole

Peroxisomes:

- Contains oxidases,
- Catabolism of H_2O_2

Mitochondria:

- Site of ATP synthesis
- Site of Krebs cycle, beta-oxidation of fatty acids, oxidative phosphorylation & acetyl CoA production

Mitochondrial DNA:

- Double stranded, circular molecule
- Inheritance is strictly maternal

Golgi complex:

- Post-translational modifications of proteins (sulfation, phosphorylation)
- Protein sorting & packaging (Secretory proteins like insulin are packed into clathrin coated vesicles)

BODY FLUIDS

Water:

- 60% of body weight (IntraCellular Fluid is 40% & ExtraCellular Fluid is 20%)
- Rest 40% of body weight is because of organic/ inorganic material (18% protein + 15% fat + 7% minerals)

Extracellular fluid:

- ECF is 20% of body weight
- Includes plasma (5% of body weight) & interstitial fluid (15% of body weight)

Body fluids:

- Sodium, chloride & bicarbonate ions are predominant in: ECF
- Intracellular fluid is rich in: Potassium
- Endolymph is rich in: Potassium
- Normal anion gap (cations - anions): 10-12 mmol/ L
- Measurement of Total body water: Tritiated water/ deuterium oxide
- Measurement of Extracellular fluid volume: Inulin, mannitol, thiocyanates
- Measurement of Plasma volume: Evans blue, RBCs labelled with phosphorous-32/ chromium-51

Terms:

- Colloid oncotic/ osmotic pressure: Pressure due to plasma colloids (albumin)
- Newtonian fluid: Velocity is constant (water)

NORMAL VALUES

Normal values:

- Normal blood volume: 5-5.5 liters (3 liters plasma + 2 liters of cell volume)
- Total plasma protein in blood is: 6.4-8.3 gm/dl
- Normal albumin: globulin ratio is: 1.8:1 to 2:1
- Na^+: 135-145 meq/l
- K^+: 3.5-5.5meq/l
- Ca^{++}: 9-11meq/l
- pH: 7.35-7.45
- PCO_2: 34-45 Hg
- PO_2: 85-100 mm Hg
- HCO_3: 25-28 meq/l
- O_2 saturation: 92-96 percent
- Normal glomerular filtration rate: 125 ml/ min
- Renal blood flow: 1200 ml/min
- Renal threshold for glucose: 180 mg/dl
- Tubular maximum for glucose: 320 mg/min

PROTEINS & THEIR HALF LIVES

Proteins:

- Albumin: 2-3 weeks
- Transferrin: 1 weeks
- Pre-albumin, retinol binding protein, Fibronectin: 2 days

CELL TRANSPORT

Passive diffusion (simple passive+ facilitated diffusions):

- Transport of a substance along the gradient, energy is not required

Simple passive diffusion:

- There is diffusion along the gradient without the requirement of carrier.
- Not rate limiting.
- Doesn't follow saturation kinetics

Primary active transport:

- Transport against gradient.
- Energy is obtained by breakdown of ATP.
- Requires transport protein
- Rate limiting and saturable

Secondary active transport:

- Energy for transport is derived from sodium gradient.
- Transport against gradient requires transport protein.
- Rate limiting and saturable

REFLEXES/ LAW'S/ RULES IN PHYSIOLOGY

Cushing's reflex:

- The reflex that tends to restore the blood flow to medulla
- By causing rise in systemic arterial pressure, slowing of respiration and reflex bradycardia in case of raised intracranial pressure.

Bainbridge reflex:

- A true reflex rather than local response to stretch
- Causes receptor mediated increase in heart rate, is abolished by bilateral Vagotomy

Starling's law:

- Within physiological limits
- Force of contraction is directly proportional to the initial length of the muscle fibres, provided conditions remain the same.

Bezold-Jarisch reflex:

- It is a coronary chemoreflex mediated by left ventricular stretch receptors that are C fibers endings
- It causes a fall in systemic arterial pressure and heart rate and apnoea followed rapid breathing.

Bohr effect:

- Effect of CO_2 in the affinity of Hemoglobin for O_2
- Shift of oxygen hemoglobin dissociation curve by change in the blood in the blood CO_2, and hydrogen ions to enhance oxygenation of blood in lungs and to enhance release of oxygen from blood in the tissue.

Haldane effect:

- Binding of oxygen with hemoglobin tends to displace CO_2 from blood
- Important in promoting carbon dioxide transport.

Herring-Breurer reflex:

- The stretch receptors in bronchi and bronchioles send inhibitory signals through vagi to inspiratory centre when the lung is overinflated.

Cushing's response:

- Onset of irregular respiration, bradycardia and final increased blood pressure with increasing intracranial tension
- Due to brain stem compression.

Landsteiner's law:

- States that if an agglutinogen is present in the red cells of the blood, the corresponding agglutinin must be absent from the plasma
- If the agglutinogen is absent, corresponding agglutinin must be present in the plasma.

Sham rage behavior:

- Physical and motor manifestation of anger seen in destruction of ventromedial hypothalamic nuclei and septal nuclei.

Muller's doctrine of specific nerve energies:

- When the nerve pathways from particular sense organs are stimulated
- The sensation evoked is that for which the receptor is specialized no matter how or where along the pathway the activity is initiated.

Weber-Fechner law:

- Interpreted signal strength = Log x stimulus intensity + constant.

II. NERVE & MUSCLE PHYSIOLOGY

ACTION POTENTIAL

Action potential:

- Due to sodium influx
- Magnitude of AP is affected by ECF Na^+

Phases:

- Resting stage
- Depolarization: Permeable to Na^+ increases
- Repolarization: K^+ efflux
- Hyperpolarization: K^+ efflux is exaggerated

RESTING MEMBRANE POTENTIAL

Resting Membrane Potential of:

- RBC: -7 mV
- Smooth muscle: -50 mV
- Nerve: -70 mV
- Cardiac muscle: -90 mV

Resting membrane potential:

- Mainly due to potassium ions
- Maintained by sodium potassium ATPase
- RMP is due to: Potassium ions
- RMP is close to isoelectric potential of: Chloride ions

NERVE CONDUCTION

Nerve conduction:

- Nerve impulse begins in axon hillock
- Conduction is faster in myelinated axons
- Impulse conduction is unidirectional as neurotransmitter substance is present in vesicles of presynaptic neurons only

MUSCLE PHYSIOLOGY

Muscles:

- Skeletal muscles: Well developed striations
- Cardiac muscles:
  - o Striations present,
  - o Functionally synctial & rhythmically contracts
- Smooth cells:
  - o No striations,
  - o Found in hollow viscera & eye

Skeletal muscle fibre:

- Sarcolemma covers muscle fibre
- Muscle fibres composed of myofibrils
- Myofibrils are made up of filaments
- Filaments contains contractile proteins
- Contractile proteins:
  - o Actin,
  - o Myosin,
  - o Tropomyosin &
  - o Troponins (type I, T & C)

Muscle contraction:

- Active sites of actin are covered by: Tropo-myosin (Troponin T binds to tropo-myosin)
- Essential for muscle contraction: Cellular calcium (Troponin C binds Ca)

Excitation-contraction coupling/ ECC:

- Calcium is agent for ECC (from sarcoplasmic retiulum)
- Calcium combines with troponin-C
- Tropomyosin leaves the actin-myosin sites
- Contraction occurs

Muscle proteins:

- Myosin: Major proteins (60%), binds to actin
- Actin: F-actin has an active site
- Tropomyosin: Covers the actin binding sites

Troponins:

- Troponin T: Binds to tropomyosin
- Troponin I: Inhibits myosin & actin interaction
- Troponin C: Binds calcium

Rheobase & chronaxie

- Rheobase: The least strength or current which excites the excitable tissue
- Chronaxie: Minimum time required to stimulate the excitable tissue when strength of the current used is double the rheobase

NERVE FIBRES

Nerve fibres & their susceptibility:

- Order of susceptibility of nerve fibres to local anaesthesia/ cocaine: Type C > type B > type A
- Order of susceptibility of nerve fibres to pressure: Type A > type B > type C
- Order of Susceptibility of nerve fibres to hypoxia: B > A > C

GOLGI TENDON ORGAN & MUSCLE SPINDLE

Golgi tendon organ

- GTO detects: Muscle tension (force generated during muscle contraction)/ inverse stretch reflex/ inverse myotactic reflex
- Impulses are transmitted by: Type Ib nerve fibres

Muscle spindle:

- It is a receptor for: Myotactic/ stretch reflex
- Peripheral zone of muscle spindle has: Actin & myosin
- 2 type of fibres
  - o Extrafusal: Innervated by alpha motor neuron
  - o Intrafusal: Innervated by gamma motor neuron

Intrafusal fibres:

- Nuclear bag fibres: Detects dynamic length (discharges most rapidly)
- Nuclear chain fibres: Static length

III. CENTRAL NERVOUS SYSTEM

EEG & SLEEP

Theta waves:

- Obtained generally in children below 5 years
- Low frequency and low voltage waves
- Frequency: 4-8/ second
- Amplitude: 10 microvolts
- Theta waves are seen in: Hippocampus

Delta waves:

- Low frequency and high amplitude
- Frequency: 1-5/sec
- Amplitude: 20-200 microV
- Common in early childhood during waking hours
- In adults, it appears mostly during sleep
- Presence of delta waves in adults during conditions other than sleep is pathological like tumour, epilepsy

REM sleep:

- Occupies 20-30% of sleeping period
- Associated with rapid conjugate movements of the eyeballs
- Though the eyeballs move, but the sleep is deep so it is called paradoxical sleep
- Dreaming/ nightmare occurs

CAUDATE NUCLEUS

Caudate nucleus:

- Elongated arch gray mass, lying medial to internal capsule
- Throughout its length, the caudate nucleus is related to lateral ventricle.
- It is the region of CNS, which degenerate in Huntington's disease

LIMBIC SYSTEM

Components of limbic system:

- Archicortical structures
- Paleocortical structures
- Juxtacortical structures
- Subcortical structures

Functions of limbic system:

- Olfaction
- Regulation of endocrine glands
- Regulation of autonomic functions (heart rate, blood pressure, body temperature)
- Regulation of food intake
- Control of circadian rhythm
- Emotions & memory (Papez circuit)

SPEECH

Primary auditory area:

- 41, 42 & Wernicke's area
- 41 & 42 are situated in anterior transverse gyrus and lateral surface of superior temporal gyrus
- Wernicke's area is in upper part of superior temporal gyrus posterior to area 41 and 42
- Primary auditory area is concerned with perception of auditory impulses, analysis of pitch and determination of intensity and source of sound.
- Areas 41 and 42 are concerned only with the perception of auditory sensation (sound).
- Wernicke area is responsible for the interpretation of auditory sensation

- Lesion in Wernicke's area results in sensory aphasia

Broca's area:

- Motor area for speech
- Includes area 44 and 45
- Present in dominant hemisphere
- Special region in premotor cortex
- Responsible for movements of tongue, lips and larynx, which are responsible for speech
- Concerned with: Word formation
- Broaca area is present in: Inferior frontal gyrus

HYPOTHALAMUS

Regulation of water balance by hypothalamus by 2 mechanisms:

- Thirst mechanism
- ADH mechanism

Thirst centre:

- Thirst center is in the lateral nucleus of hypothalmus.
- There are some osmoreceptors in the areas adjacent to this which are stimulated by increase in osmolality
- Osmolality is inverse to ECF volume
- When the ECF volume decreases, the osmolality increases
- This stimulates the supraoptic nuclei also, which secretes ADH
- Nuclei of hypothalamus controlling water balance: Supraoptic nucleus
- ADH causes retention of water by facultative reabsorption in the renal tubules

Circadian/ diurnal rhythm:

- It is regular recurrence of physiological processes or activities, which occurs in cycle of 24 hours
- Suprachiasmatic nuclei plays an important role in setting the biological clock by its connection with retina
- Nuclei of hypothalamus controlling circadian rhythm: Supra-chiasmatic nucleus

Heat gain/ production center:

- Situated in posterior hypothalamus
- Nuclei of hypothalamus controlling shivering: Posterior hypothalamus
- Stimulation of this nuclei causes shivering by stimulating primary motor center
- Removal of this nuclei causes a fall in body temperature

Other nuclei of hypothalamus:

- Lateral nucles: Feeding centre
- Ventromedial nucleus: Satiety centre

Thyroxine:

- Hormone important for cold adaptation:
- Thyroid hormone increases the heat production in the body by accelerating various cellular metabolic processes and increasing BMR.

NEUROTRANSMITTERS

Excitatory neurotransmitter in CNS:

- Glutamate (main)
- Ach
- NO
- Histamine
- Aspartate

Flight or fight response:

- Increased heart rate,
- Increased BP,
- Increased total peripheral resistance

CEREBELLUM

Comparator function:

- Cerebellum receives information from cerebral cortex and feedback information (proprioception) from muscles
- By receiving the messages from both the ends, corticocerebellum compares the cortical commands for muscular activity
- Based on impulses from cerebellum,

cerebral cortex corrects or modifies the signals to muscles, so that the movements become accurate, precise and smooth.

Functions of Vestibulocerebellum:

- Regulates tone, posture and equilibrium by receiving impulses from vestibular apparatus

Functions of Spinocerebellum:

- Regulates tone, posture and equilibrium by receiving sensory impulses from tactile receptors, proprioceptors, visual receptors and auditory receptors

Functions of Corticocerebellum/ Neocerebellum:

- Concerend with the integartion and regulation of well-coordinated muscular activities.

Effect of cerebellar lesions:

- Disturbance in tone and posture:
  - o Atonia/ hypotonia
  - o Pendular jerks
- Disturbance in equilibrium:
  - o Body sways side
  - o Staggering/ drunken-like gait
- Disturbance in movements:
  - o Ataxia (lack of coordination of movements)
  - o Asynergia
  - o Asthenia
  - o Dysmetria & past-pointing
  - o Intention tremor
  - o Nystagmus
  - o Dysarthria
  - o Adiadochokinesia

BASAL GANGLIA

Basal ganglia:

- Forms part of extrapyramidal system, which is concerned with motor activities
- Function of basal nuclei/ basal ganglia: Programming of movements
- Caudate nucleus & lentiform nuclei (corpus striatum) are a part of: Basal ganglia

Components of basal ganglia:

- Corpus striatum (caudate nucleus and lenticular nucleus)
- Substantia nigra
- Subthalamic nucleus of Luys

Functions of basal ganglia:

- Control of muscle tone
- Control of motor activity
- Control of reflex muscular activity (posture)
- Control of automatic associated movements (Facial expressions while talking)
- Role in arousal mechanism

Disorders of basal ganglia:

- Parkinson disease
- Wilson disease
- Chorea (rapid jerky movements)
- Athetosis (rhythmic and twisting movements)
- Huntington chorea
- Hemiballismus (violent involvuntary movements on one side)
- Kernicterus

Parkinson disease:

- Tremor (static/ resting/ drum-beating/ pin-rolling movements)
- Slowness of movements (bradykinesia)
- Poverty of movements (statue like, mask-like facies)
- Rigidity (lead-pipe)
- Gait (fetinating)
- Speech problem
- Dementia

CELLS OF NERVOUS SYSTEM

Cells & their functions:

- Macroglia: CNS macrophages
- Astrocytes: Maintain blood-brain barrier. Repair and scar formation
- Oligodendrocytes: Formation of myelin in CNS
- Ependymal cells: Line the ventricular system.

ROUTE OF CSF FLOW

Choroid plexus → Lateral ventricle →Foramen of Monro → Third ventricle → Aqueduct of Sylvius → Fourth ventricle → Foramina of Luschka and Magendie → Subarachnoid space → Venous outflow

REFLEXES

Reflexes & their root value:

- Ankle: S1, S2
- Knee jerk: L3, 4
- Biceps reflex: C5, 6
- Triceps jerk: C7, 8
- Radial jerk: C6
- Plantar reflex: S1,S2
- Abdominal reflex: T7, T11
- Cremasteric reflex: L1

RECEPTORS

Receptors & sensations carried:

- Free nerve endings: Detect touch and pressure
- Meissner's corpuscles: Detect movement of light touch
- Merkel's disc: Localizing touch sensations and determining texture
- Hair end organs: Detect the movement of objects on the surface of body
- Ruffini's end organs: Detect degree of joint movement
- Paccinian corpuscles: Detect tissue vibration, extremely rapid changes in mechanical state of tissue.

IV. CARDIOVASCULAR SYSTEM

CIRCULATION

Vessels:

- Resistance vessel: Arteriole
- Exchange vessel: Capillaries (maximum surface area)
- Capacitance vessel: Vein

Blood pressure:

- BP is calculated as: Cardiac output X peripheral resistance
- Small cuff, thick walled vessels & obesity will give a: High BP
- SI unit: kPa
- Korotkoffs sound: Produced by turbulent flow in the brachial artery
- Pulse pressure: SBP – DBP
- Mean arterial pressure: DBP + 1/3 (PP)

Some important terms:

- Ventricular end diastolic volume:
  - o Volume of blood in ventricular cavity at the end of atrial contraction (120 ml)
  - o Determines preload
- Ejection fraction:
  - o Ratio of stroke volume to end diastolic volume (SD/ EDV)
  - o 50-70%
- Stroke volume:
  - o Volume of blood ejected with each heart beat (CO/ HR);
  - o 70-80 ml
- Cardiac index:
  - o Cardiac output/ Body surface area;
  - o 3.2 is the normal value

CONDUCTION

Depolarization proceeds from:

- SA node → AV node → Bundle of His → Bundle branches

Order of ventricular depolarization:

- Endocardium surface of Interventricular septum (left to right)
- Ventricle from endocardium to epicardium
- Topmost portion of IV septum, base of heart & the pulmonary conus (last to be depolarized)

ECG

12 conventional ECG leads:

- 6 limb/ extremity leads
- 6 chest/ precordial leads

6 limb leads:

- 3 standard bipolar leads (I, II, III)
- 3 augmented unipolar leads (aVR, aVL and aVF)

Leads:

- Lead I: Left arm – right arm
- Lead II: Left leg – right arm
- Lead III: Left leg – left arm
- aVR: Right arm
- aVL: Left arm
- aVF: Left leg

6 chest leads:

- V1: 4th intercostal space/ ICS (right of sternum)
- V2: 4th ICS (left of sternum)
- V3: Midway between V2 & V4
- V4: Midclavicular line, 5th ICS
- V5: Anterior axillary line (same level as V4)
- V6: Mid-axillary line (same level as V4)

ECG

Components:

- P wave
- PR interval
- QRS complex
- QT interval
- T wave
- U wave

ECG (Value & coinciding event):

- P wave (0.08): Atrial depolarization
- PR interval (0.12-0.20 sec): Atrial depolarization and conduction through AV node measured from beginning of QRS complex.
- QRS duration (0.08-0.10 sec): Ventricular depolarization and atrial repolarization
- T wave: Ventricular repolarization
- U wave: Slow repolarization of papillary muscles.

CARDIAC CYCLE

Phases of cardiac cycle:

- IVC (isovolumetric contraction)
- Systolic ejection
- IVR (isovolumetric relaxation)
- Rapid ventricular filling
- Slow ventricular filling

HEART SOUNDS

1st heart sound/ S1:

- Because of closure of AV valves
- ECG: R wave
- JVP: c wave
- Starting of isovolumetric ventricular contraction

2nd heart sound/ S2:

- Due to closure of aortic & pulmonary valves
- ECG: End of T wave
- JVP: Beginning of v wave

3rd heart sound/ S3:

- Heard during early/ first rapid Ventricular filling phase
- Stretching of chordae tendinae/ papillary muscle
- ECG: Starting of p wave
- JVP: End of v wave

4th heart sound/ S4:

- Atrial contraction/ last/ rapid filling phase of ventricles
- ECG: p wave
- JVP: a wave

WAVES OF JVP

a wave:

- Due to right Atrial contraction
- Heart sound: Precedes S1

c wave:

- Due to right ventricular contraction, which pushes the tricuspid valve in right atrium
- Heart sound: After S1

v wave:

- Due to right atrial filling

x wave:

- Due to atrial relaxation (chordial pulling of tricuspid ring)
- Precedes S2

y wave:

- Due to opening of tricuspid valve
- After S2

MYOCARDIAL ACTION POTENTIAL

Phases of action potential in myocardium:

- Phase 0: Initial depolarization
- Phase 1: Initial rapid repolarization
- Phase 2: Plateau (Calcium influx)
- Phase 3: Rapid repolarization
- Phase 4: Resting potential

V. GASTROINTESTINAL TRACT

SITE OF ABSORPTION

Site of absorption of:

- Iron: Duodenum & proximal jejunum
- Calcium & folic acid: Jejunum
- Bile salts & Vitamin B_{12}: Terminal ileum

BICARBONATE

Physiology of bicarbonate:

- Secreted by: Mucosal cells of stomach & duodenum
- Action: Neutralization of acid (prevents autodigestion)
- Secretion increased by: Secretin
- Alkaline tide: Bicarbonate is released in exchange for chloride

PEPSIN

Physiology of pepsin:

- Secreted by: Chief cells in body of stomach
- Action: Digestion of proteins
- Secretion increased by: Vagal stimulation and local acid
- Hydrogen ion converts inactive pepsinogen to active pepsin

INTRINSIC FACTOR

Physiology of IF:

- Secreted by: Parietal cells in body of stomach
- Action: Required for absorption of vitamin B_{12} (extrinsic factor)
- In Pernicious anemia, there is autoimmune destruction of parietal cells

GASTRIC ACID

Physiology of HCl:

- Secreted by: Parietal/ Oxyntic cells in body of stomach
- Action: Reduces pH of stomach
- Secretion increased by: Gastrin, Acetylcholine & histamine
- Gastrinoma is a gastrin producing tumour resulting in increased gastric acid secretion & ulcer formation

GASTRIN

Physiology of gastrin:

- Secreted by: G cells in antrum of stomach
- Action:
  - o Increases secretion of gastric acid, pepsin & intrinsic factor
  - o Increases gastric motility & emptying
- Secretion increased by: Peptides & amino acids, vagal stimulation
- Gastrinoma/ Zollinger Ellison syndrome: Gastrin producing tumour

SECRETIN

Physiology of secretin:

- Secreted by: S cells of duodenum & jejunum
- Action:
  - o Increased pancreatic bicarbonate secretion (neutralization of gastric acid)
  - o Reduces gastric acid & pepsin secretion
- Secretion increased by: Presence of hydrogen ions & fatty acids in duodenum
- Most potent stimulator of secretion of secretin is: Acidic chyme

CHOLECYSTOKININ

Physiology of CCK-PZ:

- Secreted by: J cells of duodenum & jejunum
- Action:
  - o Increased pancreatic enzyme and bicarbonate secretion
  - o Increased gall bladder contraction for bile secretion
- Secretion increased by: Fatty acids, amino acids, peptides

MOTILITY

Gastric motility stimulated by:

- Gastrin
- Acetylcholine
- Distension
- Histamine
- Angiotensin

Gastric motility inhibited by:

- Fatty acids
- Acid in duodenum
- CCK
- Secretin

VI. RESPIRATORY PHYSIOLOGY

SPIROMETRY

Total lung capacity:

- Volume of air contained in the lung at the end of maximal inspiration
- 6 L (male); 4.7 L (female)
- Total lung capacity depends upon: Lung compliance

Vital capacity:

- Amount of air that can be forced out of the lungs after maximal inspiration
- 4.8 L (male); 3.6 L (female)

Tidal volume:

- Amount of air breathed in or out during normal breathing
- 500 ml (male); 390 ml (female)

Inspiratory reserve volume/ IRV:

- Air that can be taken in over and above the tidal volume

Expiratory reserve volume/ ERV:

- Maximum volume of air that can be expired over and above the tidal volume

Residual volume/ RV:

- Volume of air that remains in the lungs after forceful expiration

Inspiratory capacity:

- Maximum volume of air that can be inspired after normal tidal expiration
- IC=IRV+TV

Vital capacity:

- Maximum volume of air that can be expired after deepest possible inspiration
- VC=IRV +TV+ERV

Total lung capacity: Sum of vital capacity and residual volume

SURFACTANT

Surfactant:

- Pulmonary surfactant is secreted by: Type II pneumocytes

- Surfactant is: DPPC (Dipalmitoyl phosphatidyl choline)
- Surfactant production is accelerated by: Glucocorticoids
- Respiratory distress syndrome is due to: Deficiency of surfactant

CENTRES OF RESPIRATION

Pneumotaxic centre:

- Present in Upper Pons (dorsal)
- Inhibits respiration
- Regulates respiratory volume & respiratory rate

Apneustic centre:

- Present in Lower Pons
- Inhibits respiration
- Produces deep & prolonged inspiratory gasp

Respiratory group/ RG:

- Dorsal RG: Inspiratory
- Ventral respiratory group (active during forceful breathing): Expiratory

OXYGEN DISSOCIATION CURVE

Shift to left (oxygen remains bonded to hemoglobin):

- Increased pH,
- Decreased temperature,
- Fetal hemoglobin

Shift to right (oxygen released):

- Decreased pH,
- Increased temperature
- Increased 2,3,DPG

HYPOXIA

Hypoxic/ anoxic Hypoxia:

- Low pO_2 of the arterial blood
- Seen in high altitudes

Anemic Hypoxia:

- Arterial pO_2 is normal
- Oxygen carrying capacity of blood is low
- Seen in anemia & carbon monoxide poisoning

Stagnant/ ischemic Hypoxia:

- Normal pO_2 & normal O_2 content
- But decreased rate of blood flow to tissues
- Seen in congestive cardiac failure

Histotoxic hypoxia:

- Cells cannot utilize O_2 delivered to them
- Seen in cyanide poisoning

VII. ENDOCRINAL SYSTEM

INSULIN

Insulin Increases:

- Lipogenesis (cholesterol & triglyceride synthesis)
- Protein synthesis
- Glycolysis
- Glycogenesis
- Glucose transport (muscle, adipose tissue)

Physiology of Insulin:

- Insulin is secreted by: Beta cells of pancreas
- Insulin secretion is inhibited by: Epinephrine
- Insulin acts through: Tyrosine kinase activity
- Insulin receptor is a cell membrane receptor, a heterotetrameric glycoprotein made of 2a and 2b subunits linked by disulfide bonds; the b subunit has tyrosine kinase activity

PARATHORMONE

Effect of parathormone (produced by chief cells of parathyroid):

- Stimulates osteoclastic activity (increased bony resorption by osteoclasts)

- Augments reabsorption of calcium in DCT
- Decreased kidney reabsorption of phosphate
- Augments absorption of calcium from the gut

CALCITONIN

Effect of calcitonin (produced by chief cells of thyroid):

- Opposite to that of PTH (antagonist to PTH),
- Lowers serum calcium,
- Acts by decreasing osteoclasis (bone resorption)
- Hence human calcitonin is used in Paget's disease and osteoporosis
- Decreases proximal tubular calcium and phosphate reabsorption by direct action on kidney

Hypocalcemia:

- A decrease in concentration of free calcium ions in plasma:
    - o Increased neuromuscular irritability & tetani
    - o Chvostek's sign
- ECG finding of hypocalcemia: Lengthening of the QT interval

ANTERIOR PITUITARY

Anterior pituitary gland/ adenophysis:

- Derivative of Rathke's pouch
- Synthesize FSH, LH, ACTH, TSH, GH, prolactin
- Release of hormones is controlled by hypothalamus

POSTERIOR PITUITARY

Posterior pituitary gland/ Neurohypophysis:

- Develops from down-growth from the floor of the third ventricle (diencephalon)
- Vasopressin & oxytocin are synthesized in the hypothalamus and shipped to the posterior pituitary

THYROID

Thyroid gland:

- Produces T4 (thyroxine) and T3 (tri-iodo-thyronine)
- T4 is converted to T3 by peripheral tissue
- T3/ T4 is bounded by thyroid binding globulin/ TBG
- Free hormone is active

Regulation of thyroid hormone secretion:

- TRH (from hypothalamus) stimulates TSH (from anterior pituitary) follicular cells of thyroid.

Wolff-Chaikoff effect:

- Large doses of iodides act directly on the thyroid to reduce hormone synthesis (it produce a mild and transient inhibition of organic binding of iodide)

HORMONE RECEPTORS

Cell membrane receptors:

- cAMP pathway: Adrenaline, Calcitonin, Glucagon, TSH, FSH, LH, ACTH, PTH.
- IP3-DAG: Vasopressin, Oxytocin
- Tyrosine- kinase: Insulin, Growth hormone

Cytoplasmic receptors:

- Steroids (Glucocorticoids, Mineral-ocorticoids), Estrogen, Progesterone

Nuclear receptors:

- Thyroxine

ADRENAL CORTEX

Zones & hormone secreted:

- Zona Glomerulosa: Aldosterone
- Zona Fasciculate: Cortisol
- Zona Reticularis: Androgens

VIII. EXCRETORY SYSTEM

RENIN

Renin Angiotensin system:

- Renin released by juxtaglomerular apparatus after sensing low BP
- It converts Angiotensinogen (from liver) → Angiotensin I
- Angiotensin I → Angiotensin II by angiotensin converting enzyme (in lung capillaries)

Angiotensin II:

- Powerful vasoconstrictor
- Release of aldosterone from adrenal cortex
- Release of ADH from posterior pituitary
- Overall it causes an increase in intravascular volume à increased BP

Renin:

- Action: Converts angiotensinogen to angiotensin I
- Factors stimulating renin secretion: Low BP, Hyponatremia etc.

PARTS OF KIDNEY & THEIR FUNCTIONS

Function of proximal convoluted tubules:

- Active reabsorption of all glucose & amino acids and most of the sodium, potassium, amino acids etc.
- Passive reabsorption of urea & water

Function of Loop of Henle:

- Site of counter current multiplier (maximum reabsorption of water à concentration of urine under effect of ADH)

Thin descending limb of loop of Henle:

- Passively reabsorbs water (makes urine hypertonic)

Thick ascending limb of loop of Henle:

- Actively reabsorbs sodium, potassium & chloride (makes urine hypotonic)

Function of distal convoluted tubule:

- Actively reabsorbs sodium & chloride
- Reabsorption of calcium (under effect of parathormone)

Function of collecting tubule & duct:

- Reabsorbs sodium in exchange for secreting potassium or hydrogen (under effect of aldosterone)
- Reabsorption of water (under effect of anti-diuretic hormone)

PROXIMAL CONOVOLUTED TUBULE

Reabsorption in PCT:

- Major part of glomerular filtrate is absorbed in: PCT
- Substances completely reabsorbed in PCT: Glucose, K^+, Amino acid
- Substances partially (75-80%) reabsorbed in PCT: Sodium, Chloride Bicarbonate, Water

JUXTAGLOMERULAR APPARATUS

Parts of JGA:

- Juxtaglomerular cells (renin secreting cells in wall of afferent arteriole)
- Macula densa (modified distal convoluted epithelium)
- Granular lacis cells

CHAPTER 3

BIOCHEMISTRY

I. ENZYMES

ISO-ENZYMES

Isoenzymes:

- Physically different forms of a same enzyme which catalyze same biochemical reaction
- Creatine kinase isoenzymes:
  - o CK-1 (BB): Brain
  - o CK-2 (MB): Heart
  - o CK-3 (MM): Skeletal muscle
- Lactate dehydrogenase isoenzymes:
  - o LDH-1 (HHHH): Heart
  - o LDH-2 (HHHM): Blood (WBC)
  - o LDH-3 (HHMM): Brain, kidney, lungs & pancreas
  - o LDH-4 (HMMM): Muscle & liver
  - o LDH-5 (MMMM): Muscle & liver

CLASSES OF ENZYMES

Oxidoreductases:

- Catalyze oxidation-reductions reactions
- Examples: LDH

Transferases:

- Catalyze transfer of C-, N- or P groups
- Example: Aminotransferase

Lyase:

- Can break a bond or make a bond but without using water of ATP
- Example: Aldolase A

Ligase:

- Catalyze formation of bond by use of ATP
- Example: Pyruvate carboxylase

Hydrolase

- Use H_2O to break a bond
- Example: Urease

Isomerase:

- Interconverts isomers
- Example: Methyl malonyl CoA mutase

PARTS OF AN ENZYME

- Coenzyme is: Non protein organic compounds (all coenzyme are cofactors)
- Apoenzyme: Protein part
- Holoenzyme: Active enzyme

ENZYME INHIBITION

Competitive:

- Both inhibitor and substrate compete for the active site of enzyme
- Inhibitor binds with free enzyme, reversibly, to form enzyme-inhibitor complex, that is catalytically inactive
- Substrate cannot bind
- So a high concentration of substrate is required to offset the binding of inhibitor to the enzyme.
- So K_m increases.
- V_{max} remains same
- Inhibitor cannot bind with E-S complex

Non-competitive:

- Inhibitor and substrate have different sites of binding on enzyme.

- Inhibitor doesn't bind at the active site
- Inhibitor can bind with Enzyme-substrate/ E-S complex
- So K_m remains same
- V_{max} is lowered

II. AMINO ACID & PROTEINS

AMINO ACIDS/ AA

Important points:

- Total number of AA: 22
- 21st AA: Selenocysteine
- Essential AA: These are required in diet as they cannot be synthesized in the body
- Semi-essential AA: These are synthesized in the body but to some extent (Arginine & Histidine)
- Non-essential AA: These are not required in diet as they are synthesized in the body
- Branched chain amino acid whose metabolism is abnormal in maple syrup urine disease/ MSUD: Leucine, Isoleucine, Valine
- Most non polar amino acid is: Leucine
- Amino acid containing indole ring: Tryptophan
- Creatine is synthesized from (GAME):
  - o **G**lycine,
  - o **A**rginine,
  - o **Me**thionine
- Buffering action of blood is due to which amino acid: Histidine

ALIPHATIC AMINO ACIDS

Glycine:

- Formation of
  - o Glutathione
  - o Creatine
  - o Haem

Alanine:

- Non-essential
- Alanine forms pyruvate (glucogenic)

Valine, Leucine & Isoleucine:

- Branched chain AA
- Defect in catabolism leads to MSUD

AROMATIC AMINO ACIDS

Phenyl-alanine/ PA:

- Alanine + phenyl ring
- Essential AA

Tyrosine:

- Enzyme phenyl-alanine hydroxylase converts PA to tyrosine
- Non-essential as it can be synthesized in body from PA
- Used for synthesis of:
  - o Melanin
  - o Thyroid hormones
  - o Catecholamines
    - – Dopamine
    - – Nor-epinephrine
    - – Epinephrine

Tryptophan:

- Forms:
  - o Serotonin (5-hydroxytryptamine)
  - o Melatonin
  - o Niacin (vitamin B3)

Histidine:

- Essential but semi-essential
- Maximum buffering capacity
- Catabolic end-product is glutamate

BASIC AMINO ACIDS/ POSITIVELY CHARGED AA

Members:

- Arginine
- Lysine

  Histidine

Points:

- Arginine is most polar whereas Histidine is least polar

ACIDIC AMINO ACIDS

Members:

- Aspartate
- Glutamate

Points:

- Non-essential as they can be synthesized from TCA/ Kreb's cycle intermediates

-OH CONTAINING AMINO ACIDS

Members:

- Serine
- Threonine
- Tyrosine

SULPHUR AMINO ACIDS/ AA

Members:

- Cysteine
- Methionine

IMINO ACIDS

Proline:

- Unique structure helps proline in the fibrous structure of collagen

PROTEINS

Structure of proteins:

- Primary structure: Sequence of AA joined by peptide bond
- Secondary structure: folding of primary structure
  - o Alpha helix
  - o Beta sheet
- Tertiary structure: Single fully folded functional polypeptide chain
- Quarternary structure: Spatial relationship between individual polypeptide chains

AMINO ACID METABOLIC DEFECTS

Phenylketonuria/ PKU:

- PKU is due to deficiency of: Phenylalanine hydroxylase/ PAH
- PAH converts Pheny Alanine/ PA to Tyrosine
- Tyrosine becomes essential as it is not formed and there is excess of PA in body
- Excess PA is converted into Phenyl acetate & Phenyl pyruvate
- Mousy/ musty odour of urine (due to Phenyl acetate)
- Diagnosis:
  - o Guthrie's test for screening
  - o Urinary $FeCl_3$ test (due to Phenyl pyruvate)
- Treatment:
  - o Give Tyrosine as its not formed
  - o Lifelong restriction of PA in diet

Alkaptonuria:

- It is due to deficiency of: Homogentisate oxidase
- Defect in catabolism of tyrosine & PA
- Urine turns black on exposure to air (due to oxidation of Homogentisic acid/ HGA)
- Ochronosis: Deposition of black pigments (polymerization of HGA) in joints, collagenous tissue and cartilage
- Treatment:
  - o Vitamin C
  - o Restriction of tyrosine & PA

UREA CYCLE

Urea cycle/ UC:

- Site of UC: Mitochondria & cytoplasm
- First 2 reactions of urea cycle occur in: Mitochondria (rest in cytoplasm)
- UC occurs in liver
- Carbamoyl Phosphate Synthetase-I is the rate limiting enzyme

III. CARBOHYDRATE

CLASSIFICATION

Monosaccharide:

- One carbohydrate unit
- Examples:
  - o Glucose
  - o Fructose
  - o Galactose

Disaccharide:

- 2 carbohydrate unit
- Examples:
  - o Sucrose
  - o Maltose
  - o Isomaltose
  - o Lactose

Oligosaccharide:

- Two to ten carbohydrates units
- Examples:
  - o Maltotriose

Polysaccharide:

- More than 10 carbohydrate units
- Homopolysaccharide
  - o Glycogen
  - o Starch
  - o Cellulose
  - o Chitin
  - o Inulin
- Heteropolysaccharide
  - o Hyaluronic acid
  - o Chondroitin sulfate
  - o Dermatan sulfate
  - o Keratin sulfate
  - o Heparan sulfate
  - o Heparin

GLYCOLYSIS/ EMP PATHWAY/ EMBDEN MEYERHOFF PATHWAY

Glycoslysis:

- Occurs in all the cell of the body
- Only pathway which can occur in both aerobic as well as anaerobic condition
- Occurs in cytoplasm
- Insulin activates it
- Catabolic process
- Glycolysis is regulated at:
  - o Hexokinase
  - o Phosphofructokinase
  - o Pyruvate kinase
- 7 ATPs are obtained in aerobic glycolysis
- 2 ATPs are obtained in anaerobic glycolysis
- Tissue which depend on glucose as fuel:
  - o Brain
  - o Red blood cells
  - o Gastrointestinal tract
  - o Renal medulla
  - o Cancer cells
- Inhibitors of glycolysis:
  - o Iodoacetate
  - o Sodium fluoride
  - o Arsenate

KREB'S CYCLE/ TCA CYCLE/ CITRIC ACID CYCLE

Tricarboxylic acid cycle:

- Mature RBC lacks enzymes of: TCA/ tricarboxylic acid cycle
- First substrate of citric acid cycle is: Acetyl CoA which is derived from Pyruvate
- Substrate level phosphorylation occurs in reaction catalyzed by enzyme: Succinyl-CoA-thiokinase
- Amphibolic (both anabolic & catabolic) pathway
- Occurs in mitochondria
- Occurs in aerobic condition
- Begins & ends with oxalo-acetate
- First substance formed is Citric acid
- A total of 10 ATPs are produced per Acetyl CoA
- Inhibitors of TCA cycle:
  - o Malonate
  - o Fluoro-acetate

GLUCONEOGENESIS

Gluconeogenesis:

- Occurs from:
  - o Glycerol
  - o Alanine
  - o Lactate
  - o Pyruvate
  - o Propionic acid
- Muscle cannot make use of glycogen as they lack: G-6-Phosphatase
- Catabolic pathway
- Occurs in
  - o Liver & kidney
  - o In mitochondria & cytoplasm
- Activated by Glucagon
- Occurs in fasting state

HMP SHUNT

Hexose Mono Phosphate pathway:

- Minor pathway for production of glucose
- It is important as it produces: NADPH
- ATP produced in HMP shunt: No ATP is directly produced/ consumed
- Anabolic pathway
- Occurs in:
  - o Cytoplasm
  - o Liver, adipose tissue
- NADPH is used for:
  - o Fatty acid synthesis
  - o Steroid synthesis
- Important enzyme involved in NADPH synthesis: G6PD

GLYCOGEN STORAGE DISEASES

GST:

- Most of the diseases in this category affect glycogenolysis (breakdown of glycogen is affected)
- Enzyme deficient in von-Gierke's disease (Type I GST): Glucose-6-phosphatase deficiency (affecting liver)
- Lactic acid & hyperuricemia is a feature of: Von-Gierke's disease (GST-I)
- Muscles are not involved in: Von-Gierke's disease (GST-I)
- Hypoglycemia, non-responsive to epinephrine is a feature of: Von-Gierke's disease (GST-I)
- Enzyme deficient in Andersons disease/ Amylopectinosis (Type IV GST): Branching enzyme (affects liver, muscle & brain)
- Enzyme deficient in McArdle's disease (Type V GST): Muscle phosphorylase (affects muscle)

GALACTOS METABOLISM

Galactosemia:

- Most common (of the 3) enzyme deficient in classical type galactosemia: GALT/ Galactose-1-phosphate-uridyl transferase
- Cataract occurs because of the accumulation of: Galactilol/ Dulcitol
- Oil drop cataract
- Age of presentation is 1st week to 1st month of life
- Give lactose free diet (avoid breast feeding)

ELECTRON TRANSPORT CHAIN

ETC:

- Electron transport chain is located in: Inner mitochondrial membrane
- Requires oxygen (aerobic)
- In electron transport chain, FADH gives: 1.5 ATP
- In electron transport chain, NADH gives: 2.5 ATP
- Components:
  - o 5 protein complexes (I - V)
  - o Coenzyme Q
  - o Cytochrome C
- Cyanide inhibits:
  - o Cytochrome oxidase (inhibits electron flow)
  - o Complex IV
  - o Cellular oxidation

- Cytochrome C oxidase/ complex IV is inhibited by:
  - o Cyanide
  - o Carbon monoxide
  - o Hydrogen sulphide
- Complex III is inhibited by Phenformin (oral hypoglycemic agent)
- Uncoupler of oxidation & phosphorylation: 2, 4-Dinitrophenol/ DNP

IV. FATS & LIPIDS METABOLISM

FATTY ACIDS

Monosaturated fatty acids:

- One double bond present
- Oleic acid

Essential fatty acid/ Polyunsaturated fatty acids/ PUFAs:

- Essential in diet (as they are not synthesized in the body)
- Omega -3 category
  - o Cervonic acid
  - o Alpha-Linolenic acid
  - o Timnodonic acid
- Omega-6 category
  - o Linoleic acid
  - o Gamma-Linolenic acid
  - o Arachidonic acid
- Most essential fatty acid is: Linoleic acid (it can synthesize arachidonic acid)

CHOLESTEROL

Cholesterol synthesis:

- Acetyl CoA is the starting material
- Rate limiting enzyme in cholesterol synthesis: HMG CoA reductase
- Anabolic pathway
- Occurs in Cytoplasm
- Insulin activates it
- Bile acids are derived from: Cholesterol

FATTY ACID/ FA

Synthesis of FA:

- Synthesis of fatty acid occurs in: Cytosol
- Anabolic pathway
- Rate limiting step in fatty acid synthesis: Acetyl CoA carboxylase (contains biotin)
- Starting material: Acetyl CoA
- Activated by Insulin
- Main enzyme: FA synthase complex

Beta oxidation of fatty acids:

- Activation by Glucagon
- Occurs in:
  - o Mitochondria
  - o Liver, adipose tissues, muscles
- Occurs in starvation/ fasting state
- Catabolic pathway
- Beta-oxidation of odd chain FA leads to production of propionyl CoA
- ATP produced by beta oxidation of palmitic acid: 106 new

Minor oxidation pathways:

- Alpha oxidation occurs in peroxisomes and endoplasmic reticulum
- Omega oxidation occurs in endoplasmic reticulum

KETONE BODIES/ KB

KB:

- Ketone bodies are:
  - o Acetoacetate (primary KB)
  - o Acetone (secondary KB)
  - o Beta-hydroxyl butyrate (secondary KB; Most common)
- Rate limiting step in KB synthesis is HMG CoA synthase
- Ketone bodies are formed in which organ: Liver
- KB are produced normally in minimal amounts but this amount is significantly raised during fasting & starvation
- Ketone bodies are product of:
  - o Increased lipolysis (Fatty acids metabolism)

  - Increased acetyl CoA or decreased oxaloacetate
- Ketone bodies are normally produced from: Acetyl CoA
- 1st KB synthesized is Acetoacetate
- Ketone bodies are utilized by conversion of aceto-acetate to: Aceto-acetyl CoA
- Important feature of starvation ketosis: Ketone body formation without glycosuria

LIPOPROTEINS

Lipoproteins:

- HDL (high density)
- LDL (low density)
- VLDL (very low density)
- IDL (intermediate density)
- Chylomicron
- Most atherogenic lipoprotein: LDL (bad cholesterol)
- Lipoprotein with highest cholesterol content: LDL
- Lipoprotein with highest exogenous triglyceride content: Chylomicrons
- Lipoprotein which reverses cholesterol transport: HDL (good cholesterol)

V. NUCLEOTIDE

NUCLEOTIDE

Sugars:

- In RNA: Ribose
- In DNA: Deoxyribose

General information:

- Nucleoside: Nitrogenous base + Sugar
- Nucleotide: Nucleoside + phosphate
- Bases: Purine & Pyrimidine
- Purine:
  - Adenine (A) &
  - Guanine (G)
- Pyrimidine:
  - Cytosine (C)
  - Uracil (U) &
  - Thymine (T)
- Bases in DNA: A, G, C and T (U is absent in DNA)
- Base present only in RNA & not in DNA: U

Purines:

- Occurs mainly in liver
- 2 pathways:
  - Denovo pathway
  - Salvage pathway
- Key enzyme/ Rate limiting enzyme for de-novo synthesis pathway of purines: PRPP Glutamyl amido transferase
- Enzyme needed for salvage pathway of purines: HGPRTase
- End product of catabolism of purines in human beings: Uracil
- Reaction catalyzed by xanthine oxidase: XO converts hypoxanthine to xanthine and xanthine to uric acid

Pyrimidine:

- Rate limiting step for pyrimidine synthesis
  - Prokaryotes: Aspartate transcarbamoylase
  - Eukaryotes: Carbamoyl phosphate synthetase-II (CPS-II)

Orotic aciduria:

Type I: OPRT & decarboxylase

Type II: Due to deficiency of: OMP decarboxylase

DNA

Bases in DNA:

- Adenine (A),
- Guanine (G),
- Cytosine (C) &
- Thymine (T)

Differences b/n RNA & DNA:

- Deoxyribose sugar of DNA is replaced by a ribose moiety,
- Instead of thymine (T), Uracil (U) is present in RNA &
- Single strand in RNA & double strands in DNA

DNA REPLICATION

DNA replication:

- New synthesized strand is made in: 5′ end → 3′ end direction
- Occurs in S-phase of cell cycle
- Okazaki fragments are formed during: Replication
- Function of helicase: DNA helix separation (zip opener)
- Semiconservative in nature (one of the parenteral strand is conserved during each cycle)
- Enzymes & functions (steps):
  - o Helicase: Separates strand
  - o Topo-isomerase: Relieve supercoils
  - o Single strand DNA binding proteins: Prevent rejoining of the 2 separated strands
  - o Primase: Synthesizes primers
  - o DNA polymerase III: Synthesize both leading & lagging strands
  - o DNA polymerase I: Remove RNA primers from both leading & lagging strands
  - o DNA ligase: Acts on lagging strand

TRANSLATION

Translation:

- Protein synthesis occurs mainly in: Ribosomes
- Fidelity enzyme in protein synthesis is: Amino acyl-tRNA synthetase
- Three steps:
  - o Initiation: Initiation codon is AUG
  - o Elongation
  - o Termination: when a stop codon is encountered on mRNA, then no AA will come.

Codons:

- Codons are nucleotide triplets
- 4 nucleotide bases are employed to produce 3 base codons: A, U, C & G
- 6 characteristic of genetic code is:
  - o 1. Triplet
  - o 2. Universal
  - o 3. Non-overlapping (A single codon have 1 amino acid)
  - o 4. Degenerate (A single amino acid can have >1 representative codon)
  - o 5. Non-punctuated
  - o 6. Exhibit wobbling
- Stop codon is: Termination codon
  - o UAA
  - o UAG
  - o UGA
- Stop codons do not code for any amino acid

TECHNIQUES IN MOLECULAR BIOLOGY

Blotting types:

- Northern blot: RNA
- Southern blot: Detects DNA
- Western blot: Proteins (Antigen)

Techniques & uses:

- Microarray/ DNA chips:
  - o Detect multiple mutations, multiple gene expression analysis, global pattern of gene expression
- FISH/ fluorescent In-situ Hybridization:
  - o Detect microdeletions, amplifications, complex translocations
- Restriction Fragment Length Polymorphism/ RFLP:
  - o Detects single mutation especially affecting pallindrome
- Karyotyping:
  - o Best technique for monosomy/ trisomy
- CRISPR-Cas 9 system:
  - o Use to know the function of gene, genome editing

POLYMERASE CHAIN REACTION

PCR:

- Enzymatic DNA amplification
- In PCR, oligonucleotides build copies of the DNA using which enzyme: Heat stable polymerase (Taq1)

- Steps of PCR:
  - Denaturation: 2 strands separated
  - Annealing: Addition of primers (one for each strand)
  - Extension/ elongation: Polymerization or synthesis of DNA
- Substances required for PCR:
  - 2 Primers
  - Thermostable polymerase (taq polymerase)
  - Magnesium
  - ds-DNA
- Helpful in:
  - Prenatal diagnosis: Beta-thalassemia, PKU
  - Retroviral infections
  - TB infections
  - Detection of cancers
  - Forensic medicine

VI. VITAMINS

CLASS OF VITAMINS

Water soluble Vitamin:

- Vitamin B
- Vitamin C

Fat soluble Vitamin:

- Absorbed into intestinal lymphatics along with dietary lipids
- They cannot be excreted by kidneys
- Vitamin A, D, E & K

Functions:

- Vitamin which prevents lipid peroxidation: Vitamin E
- Vitamin needed for gamma carboxylation: Vitamin K
- Vitamin which is a post-translation modifier: Vitamin K

VITAMIN DEFICIENCIES

Features & deficient vitamins:

- Wernicke's Korsakoff syndrome is associated with deficiency of: Thiamine (B1)
- Consumption of egg (containing avidin) may lead to deficiency of: Biotin
- Methyl malonic aciduria is seen in deficiency of: Vitamin B_{12}/ extrinsic factor of castle
- Scurvy is seen in deficiency of: Vitamin C

ENZYMES & VITAMINS

Enzyme & related vitamins:

- Alpha-keto glutarate dehydrogenase is associated with: Thiamine (B1)
- RBC Transketolase is associated with: Thiamine (B1)
- **P**yruvate **c**arboxylase is associated with (PCB): **B**iotin
- **A**mino**t**ransferases is associated with (ATP): **P**yridoxine

VII. HEMOGLOBIN

Haem:

- Present in haemoglobin, myoglobin & cytochromes.
- 'Haem' in haemoglobin is bonded to which amino acid: E7-Histidine
- Rate limiting step in haem synthesis is ALA synthase

Haem catabolism:

- Occurs in spleen, bone marrow (macrophages of reticuloendothelial system)
- Steps:
  - Bilirubin formation
  - Hepatic uptake of bilirubin
  - Bilirubin conjugation
  - Disposal of bilirubin

Haemoglobin:

- Iron in haemoglobin is present in: Ferrous (Fe^{2+}) state
- Iron in haemoglobin is held by: Polar bonds
- Alpha2, Gamma2 is: Hb fetal

CHAPTER 4

PATHOLOGY

I. GENERAL PATHOLOGY

CALCIFICATION

Dystrophic calcification:

- Occurs in dying/ non-viable tissues
- Calcium levels are normal
- Seen in caseous necrosis, liquefactive necrosis, atherosclerosis, damaged heart valves, psammoma bodies

Metastatic calcification:

- Seen in normal tissues
- Hypercalcemic state
- Seen in interstitial tissues of vessels, kidneys, lungs and gastric mucosa

NECROSIS

Fibrinoid necrosis:

- Seen in arteries, arterioles or glomerular capillaries damaged by autoimmune diseases

Fat necrosis:

- Necrosis in adipose tissue
- Induced by lipases
- Acute pancreatitis
- Trauma to adipose tissue of breast

Caseous necrosis:

- Seen in TB, fungal granuloma
- Tissue appears cheesy
- Granular material surrounded by epitheloid cells & multinucleated giant cells

Liquefactive necrosis:

- Seen in brain abscess
- Tissue is liquefied because of enzymatic action

Coagulative necrosis:

- Seen in myocardium, kidneys, liver, spleen
- MC type
- Caused by ischemia/ infarct

CELL INJURY

Features of irreversible injury:

- Cell membrane rupture
- Caspases activation
- Pyknosis (nuclear condensation)
- Karyolysis (loss of nuclear chromatin)
- Karyorrhexis (nuclear fragmentation)
- Amorphous densities in mitochondria

Apoptosis:

- Programmed cell death
- Lack of inflammation
- Mitochondria plays an important role
- Seen during embryogenesis
- Hormone dependent involution of endometrium and prostate

Morphology in apoptosis:

- Cell shrinkage
- Chromatin condensation followed by fragmentation
- Formation of cytoplasmic blebs & apoptotic bodies

Pro-apoptotic factors:

- p53
- Caspases

Anti-apoptotic factors:

- Bcl-2
- Bcl-x

HYPER SENSITIVITY REACTIONS

Type IV:

- Delayed hypersensitivity
- Cell mediated reaction
- Mantoux test
- Tuberculoid leprosy
- Contact dermatitis

Type III:

- Immune complex deposition
- Antigen antibody complex activates complement
- Acute serum sickness
- SLE
- Arthus reaction

Type II:

- Cytotoxic cytolytic reaction
- Antibody mediated (IgM, IgG)
- Transfusion reaction
- Erythroblastosis fetalis
- Goodpasture syndrome
- Myasthenia gravis

Type I:

- Anphylactic reaction
- Mediated by IgE
- Atopic asthma
- Angioedema
- Allergic rhinitis

AMYLOIDOSIS

Amyloidosis:

- Medullary Ca thyroid: A-Cal
- Senile cardiac: ATTR/ AF
- Hemodialysis associated: Abeta2 microglobulin
- Secondary amyloidosis: AA
- Primary amyloidosis: AL (light chain)

GENETICS

Autosomal dominant:

- Defect in structural gene
- One dominant mutant gene (A) is required to express the disease
- Heterozygotes (Aa) manifest the disease
- Offspring of an affected parent have 50% chances of being affected

Autosomal recessive:

- Due to enzyme deficiencies
- To express the disease, individual must be homozygous for the mutant recessive gene (aa)
- Heterozygotes (Aa) are asymptomatic carriers
- Both parents must be heterozygous (Aa) to transmit the disease

X-linked recessive:

- No male to male transmission
- Condition is transmitted by carrier women
- Affected males have normal sons and carrier daughter

X-linked dominant:

- All children of the affected homozygous females are affected
- Females pass the trait to half their sons and half their daughters
- All daughters of the affected males are affected, but none of their sons

IMMUNOGLOBULINS

IgM:

- Made of 5 monomeric Ig subunits
- Maximum molecular weight
- Primary immune response
- Intravascular
- Activates complement via classical pathway

IgG:

- 80% (most abundant)
- Crosses placenta
- Secondary immune response
- Opsonizes bacteria
- Activates complement via classical pathway

IgA:

- Secretory antibody
- Key defense for mucosal surfaces
- Activates complement via alternate pathway

COMPLEMENT

Complement system:

- Classical complement pathway is initiated by antigen-antibody complexes (IgG & IgM)
- Alternate complement pathway is initiated by bacterial cell wall (IgA complexes)
- Central process in complement pathway is conversion of C3 to C3b

II. CARDIOVASCULAR SYSTEM PATHOLOGY

VASCULAR SYSTEM PATHOLOGY

Temporal arteritis:

- Large & medium arteries (carotids & temporal)
- Segmental granulomatous inflammation
- Scalp tenderness (MC presenting symptom)
- Jaw claudication (pain on chewing/ speaking): Pathognomonic
- Severe headache (temporal)
- Polymyalgia rheumatica: Shoulder
- Thickened, tender, nodular, superficial temporal artery
- AION (altitudinal visual field defect)
- Temporal artery biopsy is diagnostic
- Fellow eye may be involved (30%)

Atherosclerotic aneurysm:

- Occur in the abdominal aorta between the renal arteries and the iliac bifurcation
- Destruction of underlying tunica media, resulting in weakening of vessel wall

Syphilitic aneurysm:

- Cor bovinum: Heart enlargement because of aortic incompetency when the aortic valve is involved
- Limited to thoracic aorta
- Intimal surface is wrinkled (tree-bark calcification)
- Seen in tertiary syphilis

CARDIAC PATHOLOGY

Rheumatic heart disease:

- Consequence of pharyngeal infection with GABHS (group A beta-hemolytic strepto-cocci)
- Type II hypersensitivity reaction
- Aschoff bodies: Pathognomonic
- MacCallum's plaques (left atrium)
- Antischkow's mycocytes (histiocytes)

Acute endocarditis:

- Large vegetations on previously normal valves
- MC caused by staph aureus
- Onset is rapid

SABE:

- mall vegetations in congenitally abnormal/ diseased valve
- Caused by streptococcus viridans (organism of low virulence)
- Insidious in onset
- Sequel of dental procedure

Clinically:

- Mitral valve is MC involved
- Tricuspid valve in I/V drug abusers
- Roth spots
- Osler's node
- Janeway lesions
- Splinter hemorrhages

MYOCARDIAL INFARCTION

MI changes:

- 2-3 hours: Waviness of myocardial fibres
- 4-12 hours: Coagulation necrosis, early neutrophilic infiltrate
- 18-24 hours: Continuing coagulation necrosis, pyknosis
- 24-72 hours: Total loss of nuclei & striations, dense neutrophilc infiltrate
- 3-7 days: Macrophage & mononuclear infiltration, fibrovascular response begins
- 10-21 days: Prominent granulation tissue
- 6 weeks: Fibrosis

III. NERVOUS SYSTEM PATHOLOGY

MENINGITIS

CSF findings in pyogenic meningitis:

- Increased protein,
- Decreased sugar Raised: Neutrophils

Features of tubercular meningitis:

- Increased protein,
- Decreased sugar,
- Increased lymphocytes

CNS TUMOURS

MC primary brain tumour:

- Adults: Glioma
- Children: Pilocytic astrocytoma

Secondaries:

- MC brain tumour in adults: Secondaries
- MC from lung carcinoma
- Malignant melanoma has greatest tendency to metastasize to the brain

Glial tumours:

- MC type of glial tumours: Astrocytoma
- Other glial tumours: Oligodendroglioma, ependymoma, choroid plexus tumour

Pilocytic astrocytoma:

- Low grade
- Benign & well circumscribed
- Good prognosis
- MC in posterior fossa
- Rosenthal fibers seen

Neuroblastoma:

- Associated with N-myc oncogene, phaeochromocytoma, neurofibromatosis
- MC tumour of adrenal medulla
- Abdominal mass, less likely hypertension
- Urinary Vanilyl Mandelic acid

Craniopharyngioma:

- Derived from Rathke's pouch
- Can cause bitemporal hemianopia (and hence confused with pituitary adenoma)
- MC childhood supratentorial tumour
- Enamel like calcification is common

BERRY ANEURYSM

Berry aneurysm:

- Associated with Autosomal Dominant Polycystic Kidney Disease/ ADPKD, Marfans syndrome, hypertension
- Occurs at the bifurcation in the Circle of Willis (MC at bifurcation of the anterior communicating artery)
- Results in hemorrhagic stroke/ Subarachnoid hemorrhage

IV. ABDOMINAL PATHOLOGY

HEPATITIS

Mallory bodies are seen in:

- Primary biliary cirrhosis,
- Alcoholism
- ICC (Indian childhood cirrhosis)
- HCC (hepatocellular Ca)
- Wilson disease

Interpretation of serological test of HBV:

- Acute HBV infection: HBsAg & IgM-anti-HBc +
- Chronic HBV infection: HBsAg & IgG-anti-HBc +
- High infectivity: HBeAg +
- Low infectivity: Anti-HBeAg +
- Immunity after vaccination: Anti-HBs +

CIRRHOSIS

Micronodular cirrhosis:

- Nodules <3 mm
- ICC (Indian childhood cirrhosis)
- Secondary biliary cirrhosis
- Haemochromatosis

Macronodular cirrhosis:

- >3 mm
- Post-necrotic
- Wilson disease

Mixed nodular cirrhosis:

- Alcohol
- Tyrosinemia
- Alpha-1-Anti-Trypsin deficiency

V. GASTROINTESTINAL TRACT PATHOLOGY

GIT PATHOLOGY

Squamous cell esophageal Ca:

- Alcohol
- Smoking
- Chronic achalasia
- Plummer vinson syndrome
- Tylosis (palmo-plantar hyperkeratosis) etc.

Ca esophagus:

- Worldwide:
  - o Squamous cell Ca is MC
  - o Affects upper 2/3rd
- In Western world:
  - o Adenocarcinoma is MC
  - o Affects lower 1/3rd

Gastrointestinal stromal tumour/ GIST:

- MC in stomach (66%)
- Originates from Interstitial cell of Cajal
- Most GIST stain positively for CD117 (part of KIT protein)
- High CD117 = High malignant potential

Peutz Jegher's syndrome:

- Inherited as autosomal dominant
- Jejunal hamartomas (juvenile polyps) plus muco-cutaneous melanin depsoits
- Malignancy very rare

NF-1/ Von Recklinghausen's disease:

- More prevalent
- Chromosome 17
- Increased risk of pheochromocytomas, juvenile myelo-monocytic leukemia
- Triad:
  - o Mulptiple cutaneous neurofibromatosis
  - o Café au lait spots (pigmented skin lesions) &
  - o Pigmented iris hamartomas

INFLAMMATORY BOWEL DISEASE

Crohn's disease:

- Distal ileum MC involved
- Skip lesions
- Transmural involvement
- Granulomas
- Creeping fat
- ASCA (antiyeast Saccharomyces cerevicae antibody) frequently positive
- X-ray:
  - o Cobblestoning of mucosa
  - o Strictures
  - o String sign & comb sign on barium swallow
- Complications:
  - o Abscess formation,
  - o Fistula
  - o Malabsorption

VI. HAMETOLOGICAL PATHOLOGY

ANEMIA

Sickle cell anemia:

- AR (autosomal recessive)
- HbS (heterozygotes) are protected from malaria
- Normocytic normochromic anemia
- Howell Jolly bodies, target cells
- Cholelithiasis
- MC feature in children: Bone pain
- Autosplenectomy

Hereditary spherocytosis:

- AD inheritance
- Massive splenomegaly, anemia, gall stones, jaundice
- Raised osmotic fragility
- Splenectomy is done

Aplastic anemia:

- Pancytopenia
- Caused by radiation, drugs, viruses, Fanconi anemia, benzene
- Severe anemia, neutropenia and thrombocytopenia with normal cell morphology
- For mild cases, RBCs and platelet transfusion

LEUKEMIA

FAB classification of AML:

- M0: Minimally differentiated AML
- M1: AML without differentiation

M2:

- AML with maturation
- MC type (30%)
- Auer rods +

M3:

- Acute promyelocytic leukemia/ APML
- Multiple Auer rods/ cell
- t(15;17)
- DIC

M4:

- Acute myelomonocytic leukemia (Naegeli type)
- NSE +ve

M5:

- Acute monocytic leukemia (Schilling type)
- Non-Specific Esterase/ NSE +ve

M6:

- Acute erythroleukemia (DiGuglielmo's disease)
- Bizarre multi-nucleated erythroblasts predominate (>50%)

M7:

- Acute megakaryocytic leukemia
- Associated with Down syndrome

CML:

- Middle aged adults are affected
- Chronic phase: Stable for several years
- Blast crisis: Accelerates into CML
- t(9;22) Philadelphia chromosome; bcr-abl fusion gene
- Weight loss, priapism, splenomegaly, anemia, sternal tenderness, painless lymphadenopathy
- Increased WBC (mainly neutrophils)
- Decreased Leucocyte alkaline phosphatase

Multiple myeloma:

- Monoclonal plasma cell cancer, producing large amount of IgG and IgA
- Back pain
- Hypercalcemia
- Anemia
- Primary amyloidosis
- Punched out ostelytic lesions
- M spike (monoclonal Ig spike) on serum protein electrophoresis
- Bence Jence proteins on urine protein electrophoresis
- Rouleaux formation
- Beta2 microglobulin (prognosis)

LYMPHOMA

Hodgkin's lymphoma:

- Bimodal distribution
- Associated with EBV
- Single group of nodes (cervical)
- Spreads centrifugally
- Reed Sternberg cells (B cell origin, owl eyes)
- B features (constitutional): Pel Ebstein fever, night sweats, weight loss

Non-Hodgkin's lymphoma:

- Widespread disease, multiple peripheral nodes
- Associated with: H pylori (MALToma), HTLV (T cell lymphoma), HIV (CNS lymphoma), EBV (Burkitt's lymphoma)

Burkitt's lymphoma:

- EBV
- B cell type
- t(8;14)
- MC in children
- c-myc gene
- Starry sky appearance

VII. EXCRETORY SYSTEM PATHOLOGY

Renomegaly:

- Diabetic nephropathy (finally shruken kidney),
- Amyloidosis,
- Polycystic kidney disease
- Hydronephrosis

Contracted kidney:

- Chronic glomerulonephritis,
- Chronic pyelonephritis
- Benign nephrosclerosis
- Myeloma kidney
- Diabetes mellitus

Flea bitten kidney:

- Malignant hypertension,
- Acute post streptococcal glomerulonephritis
- RPGN
- HUS
- TTP

GLOMERULOPATHIES

MCD/ Nil deposit disease/ lipoid nephrosis:

- MC cause of nephrotic syndrome in children
- Cause: Idiopathic (MC), Drugs (Rifampin, NSAIDS)
- T cell mediated altered capillary charge of podocyte integrity
- LM (light microscopy): Normal
- EM (electron microscopy): Loss of foot processes

PSGN/ acute diffuse proliferative GN:

- Nephritic syndrome
- RBC casts (most specific)
- Cause: Leprosy, bacterial endocarditis, Post-streptococcal (2/3rd cases)
- Immune complexes trapping
- LM: Diffuse proliferation/ endocapillary proliferation
- EM: Subepithelial deposits/ humps (lumpy bumpy deposits)
- IFM (Immuno-fluorescence microscopy): Irregular deposits of IgG + C3

MGN:

- MC cause of nephrotic syndrome in adults
- Cause: SLE, HBV, HCV
- Immune complex deposits (local)
- LM: Diffuse thickening of glomerular basement membrane
- EM: Sub-epithelial spikes & dome pattern
- IFM: Granular deposits of $C_{5b\text{-}9}$

MPGN/ mesangiocapillary GN:

- Type I is nephrotic syndrome
- Type I is immune complex disease (70%)
- LM: Split/ double counter tram track GBM, membranous thickening
- IFM: IgG + C3 deposits

RPGN/ crescentic GN:

- Nephritic syndrome
- Type I: Anti-GBM antibodies
- Type II: Immune complex
- LM: Crescents in type I
- IFM: Linear deposits of IgG + C3 in type I, anti-GBM antibody in type I (Goodpasture syndrome)

NEPHROTIC SYNDROME

Features:

- Proteinuria (>3.5 gb/ 1.73 m^2 BSA), hypoalbuminemia (<2.5 g/ dL),
- Hyperlipidemia/ hypercholesterolemia (>200 mg%)
- Edema (MC sign)

NEPHRITIC SYNDROME

Features:

- Oliguria
- Hematuria
- Edema
- +/- uremia,
- ARF &
- Hypertension

VIII. RESPIRATORY SYSTEM PATHOLOGY

ASTHMA

Types:

- Intrinsic asthma: Aspirin, cold, exercise
- Extrinsic asthma: Type I hypersensitivity reaction

Sputum findings:

- Curschmann's spirals: Whorled mucus plugs
- Charcot-Leyden crystals: Crystalloid debris of eosinophil membranes

Sampter's triad:

- Hypersensitivity to aspirin,
- Nasal allergy/ polyposis and
- Bronchial asthma

CHRONIC BRONCHITIS

Features:

- Blue bloaters
- Persistent cough with sputum production for at least 3 months in at least 2 consecutive years
- Chronic airway irritation
- Mucus hypersecretion
- Mucus gland hypertrophy
- Goblet cell metaplasia
- Reid index (gland/ wall) is used for:
  - Chronic bronchitis
  - Normal: 0.44
  - Chronic bronchitis: 0.52

EMPHYSEMA

Features:

- Pink puffer
- Abnormal & permanent dilatation of air spaces distal to the terminal bronchioles
- Excess activity of elastase & protease
- Destruction of alveolar walls

SARCOIDOSIS

Kveims test:

- Most specific test
- Involves intradermal injection of tissue from spleen/ lymph node of a patient with sarcoidosis
- Area is biopsied 4-6 weeks after injection
- Histologically examined for non-caseating grauloma

Features of sarcoidosis:

- May lead to End stage lung disease (15-30% cases);
- 65-70% recover with minimum or no residual manifestation &

- Epitheloid cells with no caseation
- Granuloma contain inclusions like:
  - o Asteroid bodies
  - o Schaumann bodies

SILICOSIS

Features:

- Can acquire pulmonary TB (silico-TB)
- Chest X-ray shows egg shell calcification & snow storm appearance
- Results because of prolonged inhalation of silica (crystalline quartz)

IX. ENDOCRINE SYSTEM PATHOLOGY

THYROID

Papillary Ca:

- MC (80%)
- Lymphatic spread (slow & late)
- Best prognosis
- Radiation induced
- May arise in thyroglossal cyst
- Psammoma bodies
- Orphan Anne eyed nuclei
- Euthyroid
- Metastatic cervical node with occult primary
- Age: 42 years
- Female: Male: 2:1

Medullary Ca thyroid/ MTC:

- Uncommon
- Earliest lymphatic spread
- Hematogenous spread also
- Familial MTC are associated with MEN IIA & IIB
- Hyaline amyloid stroma
- Secrete calcitonin

X. INFECTIOUS DISEASES

HIV

Hallmark of HIV:

- Profound immunodeficiency,
- Quantitative & qualitative deficiency of CD4+ helper or inducer T cells
- CD4+ cells are destroyed by apoptosis
- CD4+ T cell count is the best indicator of the immediate state of the immunologic competence of the patients with HIV infection

AIDS related neoplasm:

- Kaposi sarcoma,
- B cell non-Hodgkin's lymphoma,
- Primary lymphoma of brain

HIV stages:

- Acute infection
- Seroconversion
- PGL/ persistent generalized lymphadeno-pathy
- ARC/ AIDS related complex
- AIDS/ acquired immunodeficiency syndrome

CHAPTER 5

PHARMACOLOGY

I. GENERAL PHARMACOLOGY

Pharmacokinetics:

- It is the study of "what the body does to a drug"
- It is a quantitative study of drug movement in through & out of the body
- This refers to movement of the drug in and alteration of the drug by the body. It includes
  - o Absorption
  - o Distribution
  - o Binding/ localization/ storage
  - o Biotransformation and
  - o Excretion of the drug

Pharmacokinetics considerations:

- Route of administration
- Dose
- Latency of onset
- Time of peak action
- Duration of action
- Frequency of administration

Therapeutic window phenomenon:

- Optimal effect is exerted only over a narrow range of plasma drug concentration
- Between minimal therapeutic effect & the dose which produces maximal acceptable adverse effect
- E.g. TCA, clonidine, glipizide

Therapeutic index:

- Toxic dose/ Therapeutic dose
- Median lethal dose/ Median effective dose
- LD_{50}/ ED_{50}

Drug efficacy:

- Maximal effect that a drug may elicit
- Upper limit of DRC (dose-response curve)
- Morphine produces a degree of analgesia NOT obtainable with any dose of aspirin – Morphine is more efficacious than aspirin

Drug potency:

- Amount of drug required to produce a certain response
- Factor in choosing the dose of a drug
- Position of DRC on the dose axis
- More rightward = Lower potency
- 10 mg of morphine = 100 mg of pethidine as analgesic. Morphine is 10 times more potent than pethidine

BA:

- Bioavailability/ BA by intravenous route is: 100%
- Fraction of drug that reaches the systemic circulation in the unchanged form

Pro-drugs:

- Enalapril → Enalaprilat
- Levodopa → Dopamine
- Prednisone → Prednisolone
- Sulfasalazine → 5-ASA

Zero order reaction/ Capacity limited elimination/ Michaelis- Menten elimination:

- Constant AMOUNT is excreted,
- Clearance/ CL decreases with increase in concentration
- Rate of elimination INDEPENDENT of plasma concentration &

- Variable $t_{1/2}$
- E.g. Ethyl alcohol

First order ® zero order kinetics:

- Higher doses
- Plasma concentration increases disproportionately with increase in dose
- E.g. Phenytoin, Warfarin

First order reaction:

- Constant FRACTION of drug is eliminated,
- CL remains constant
- Rate of elimination is directly DEPENDENT on plasma concentration &
- $t_{1/2}$ is constant

Drug absorption:

- Basic drugs (morphine, quinine) are absorbed from: Proximal intestine (duodenum)
- Acidic drugs (salicylates, barbiturates) are predominantly unionized in the acid gastric juice and are absorbed from stomach

Microsomal enzymes:

- Located on SER
- Liver, kidney, intestinal mucosa & lungs
- Mono-oxygenase, cytochrome-P450 etc.
- Catalyze most of the oxidations, reductions, hydrolysis and glucuronide conjugation

Acetylation:

- Compounds with amino/ hydrazine residues are conjugated with the help of acetyl coenzyme-A
- Rate of acetylation shows genetic polymorphism (slow & fast acetylators)

Extra-pyramidal side-effects:

- Drugs causing extra-pyramidal side effects:
  - o Haloperidol,
  - o Levodopa
- Parkinsonism:
  - o Acute muscular dystonia: Bizarre muscle spasms
  - o Akathisia: Restlessness
  - o Malignant Neuroleptic syndrome: Rigidity, hyperthermia
  - o Tardive dyskinesia: Purposeless involuntary facial & limb movements

FIRST PASS METABOLISM

First pass/ presystemic metabolism:

- Metabolism of a drug during its passage from the site of absorption into systemic circulation
- Orally absorbed drugs → drug metabolizing enzymes in the intestinal wall & liver (through portal vein)
- Rectal route

FPM is avoided by administering the drug through:

- Sublingual
- Transdermal
- Parenteral routes

Drugs with HIGH first pass metabolism/ FPM:

- High oral dose:
  - o Beta blockers (propranolol)
  - o Salbutamol
- Not given orally:
  - o Lignocaine
  - o Isoprenaline

PHASES OF CLINICAL TRIALS

Phase I:

- Human pharmacology & safety
- Administration carried out by highly qualified clinical pharmacologists/ physician
- In a setting where all vital functions are monitored
- Emergency resuscitative facilities are available
- 20-80 Subjects (healthy mostly)
- Starting with the lowest estimated dose
- Emphasis is on safety, tolerability, and to detect any potentially dangerous effects on vital functions

Phase II:

- Therapeutic exploration & dose ranging
- Conducted by physician who are trained as clinical investigators
- 100-500 patients selected
- Primary aim is to establishment of therapeutic efficacy, dose range & ceiling effect in controlled setting
- Drug may be dropped if desired level of clinical efficacy is NOT obtained

Phase III:

- Therapeutic confirming/ Comparison
- Randomized double blind comparative trials
- 500-3000 patients
- Several physicians (specialist in treating the target disease)
- Aim is to establish the value of the drug in relation to existing therapy
- A 'NDA' is submitted to the licensing authority for permission

Phase IV:

- Post marketing surveillance/ studies
- After the drug has been marketed for general use
- Practicing physicians are identified through whom
- Data is collected on structured proforma
- About efficacy, acceptability & adverse effects of the drug
- Patient number is much larger
- Idiosyncratic/ uncommon adverse effects or those which occurs on long term use & unsuspected drug interactions are detected

Summary:

- I: Human safety
- II: Drug efficacy
- III: Comparison
- IV: Side effects/ interactions

Phase 0/ Microdosing study:

- Strategy developed to reduce down the cost and time of the drug development process
- Very low doses (1/100th of the estimated human dose are administered to healthy volunteers)

Clinical trial:

- It is a prospective ethically designed investigation in human subjects to objectively discover/ verify/ compare the results of two or more therapeutic measures (drugs)

II. DRUGS ACTING ON AUTONOMIC NERVOUS SYSTEM

Atropine:

- Uses of atropine (more potent action on heart, bronchial muscles & intestines):
- Organophosphate poisoning
- Early Mushroom/ Inocybe poisoning
- Treating brady-arrhythmias & partial heart block (selected cases)
- Pre-anaesthetic medications (reduces secretions)
- Treatment of iritis, iridocyclitis, choroiditis, keratitis & corneal ulcer

ADRENERGIC SYSTEM

Functions of alpha-1 receptors:

- Genitourinary smooth muscle contraction
- Vasoconstriction
- Gland – secretion
- Gut – relaxation
- Alpha1 agonist:
  - Phenylephrine
  - Methoxamine
- Alpha1 blockers:
  - Prazosin
  - Tamsulosin

Functions of alpha-2 receptors:

- Inhibition of transmitter release
- Vasoconstriction
- Decreased central sympathetic flow
- Alpha2 agonist:

- o Decreased central sympathetic flow
- o Clonidine
- o Methyldopa
- Alpha2 blockers:
  - o Yohimbine
  - o Mirtazapine (antidepressant)
  - o Rauwolscine

Beta1 agonist:

- Isoproterenol (beta1 = beta2)
- Dobutamine (beta1 > beta2)
- Beta1 blocker:
  - o Acebutolol
  - o Atenolol
  - o Betaxolol
  - o Bisoprolol
  - o Esmolol
  - o Metoprolol

Beta2 agonist:

- Salbutamol,
- Salmeterol,
- Terbutaline
- Ritodrine

Beta1 & Beta2 blocker:

- Dilevelol
- Labetalol
- Carvedilol (alpha1, beta1, beta2 blocker)

Esmolol:

- Shortest acting beta blocker (10 minutes)
- Action disappears 15-20 minute after terminating I/V infusion
- Uses:
  - o To terminate SVT
  - o Episodic atrial fibrillation/ flutter

III. AUTACOIDS

SEROTONIN RECEPTORS

5HT 1A agonist:

- 5-HT 1A: Present in hippocampus
- Buspirone (antianxiety)

5HT 1B agonist:

- Constricts cranial blood vessels
- Sumitriptan (migraine)

5HT 4 agonist:

- Mediates intestinal secretion,
- Augmentation of peristalsis
- Cisapride
- Renzapride (increases gastric motility)

5HT 2A antagonist:

- Post-junctional receptor mediating direct actions of 5-HT like vascular & visceral smooth muscle contraction, platelet aggregation, neuronal activation in brain
- Cyproheptadine
- Ketanserin

5HT 2A/2C antagonist:

- Clozapine

5HT 3 antagonist:

- Depolarizes neurons by gating cation channels; elicits reflex effects of 5-HT: emesis, gut peristalsis, bradycardia
- Ondansetron

PROSTAGLANDIN

PGE1:

- Misoprostol: Treatment of NSAID induced ulcer
- Alprostadil:
  - o Maintains ductus arteriosus
  - o Impotence

PGE2:

- Dinoprostone: Induction/ augmentation of labor, midterm abortion

PGF 2alpha:

- Latanoprost/ Travopost/ Bimatoprost: Treatment of glaucoma (lowers intraocular tension by enhancing uveo-oscleral and trabecular outflow)
- Latanoprost are now the first line drugs fro wide angle glaucoma

PGI2:

- Epoprostenol: Prevent platelet aggregation & damage during hemodialysis

IV. DRUGS RELATED TO ENDOCRINE SYSTEM

CORTICOIDS

Aldosterone:

- Maximum mineralo-corticoid activity is shown by: Aldosterone
- The principal mineralocorticoid action is enhancement of sodium reabsorption in the distal convoluted tubule in kidney.
- There is associated increase in K^+ and H^+ excretion

Glucocorticoid:

- Maximum gluco-corticoid activity is shown by:
  - o Dexamethasone,
  - o Betamethasone (Zero mineralocorticoid)
- Glucorticoid inhibit glucose utilization by peripheral tissues.
- This along with increased glucose release from liver results in hyperglycemia, resistance to insulin and a diabetes-like state
- They also cause protein breakdown and amino acid mobilization from peripheral tissues.
- This is responsible for side effects like muscle wasting, lympholysis, loss of osteoid from bone and thinning of skin.
- Subcutaneous tissue over extremities loses fat which is deposited over face, neck and shoulder producing 'moon face', 'fish mouth' and 'buffalo hump'.
- Glucocorticoids inhibit intestinal absorption and enhance renal excretion of calcium.
- Loss of osteoid indirectly results in loss of calcium from bone.
- Secretion of gastric acid and pepsin is increased – may aggravate peptic ulcer
- Irrespective of the type of injury or insult, the attending inflammatory response is suppressed by glucorticoids.
- This is the basis of most of their clinical uses.
- Glucocorticoids impair immunological competence.
- They suppress all types of hypersensitization and allergic phenomena.

Flutamide:

- Use of flutamide (non-steroidal androgen receptor antagonist with no hormonal activity): Metastatic prostate cancer (along with GnRH agonists)
- Flutamide is used in conjunction with GnRH agonist (to suppress LH and testosterone secretion) or after castration to block the residual action of adrenal androgens as combined androgen blockade (CAB) therapy of metastatic carcinoma prostrate

Finasteride:

- MOA of finasteride is: Selective 5-alpha reductase inhibitor which converts testosterone into more active DHT responsible for androgen action in many tissues including the prostrate gland and hair follicles)
- It is relatively selective for 5-alpha-reductase type 2 isoenzyme which predominates in male urogenital tract.
- Uses of finasteride: BPH
- Treatment with finasteride has resulted in decreased prostate size and increased peak urinary flow rate in nearly 50% patients with symptomatic benign hypertrophy of prostrate

Clomiphene:

- Anti-estrogen drug is: Clomiphene
- It binds to both estrogen receptors (ER-alpha and ER-beta) and acts as pure estrogen antagonist in all human tissues.

- It induces Gn secretion in women by blocking estrogenic feedback inhibition of pituitary.
- The amount of LH/ FSH released at each secretory pulse is increased. In response, the ovaries enlarge and ovulation occurs.

Tamoxifen:

- MOA of tamoxifen: Oral Selective Estrogen Receptor Modulator (SERM)

It has a complex action

- Acts as potent estrogen antagonist in breast carcinoma cells, blood vessels and at some peripheral sites, but as partial agonist in uterus, bone, liver and pituitary.
- Till recently tamoxifen has been the standard hormonal treatment of breast cancer in both pre- and post-menopausal women, but aromatase inhibitors (Letrozole) have now gained prominence.

V. ANTIDIABETIC DRUG

Biguanides:

- Effect of metformin (biguanide) on glucose metabolism:
  - o Overcome insulin resistance
  - o Enhances insulin mediated glucose uptake and disposal in skeletal muscle & fat (Increased glycolysis) &
  - o Decreased hepatic gluconeogensis & glucose output from liver
- Special feature of metformin:
  - o It does not cause weight gain (so particularly used in obesity; obesity is NOT a contraindication)
  - o Does NOT cause hypoglycemia (non-hypoglycemic)
- Feared complication of metformin: Lactic acidosis (More with phenformin & banned in India since 2003 for this particular side effect)
- Metformin is C/I in:
  - o Hypotensive states
  - o Heart failure
  - o Severe respiratory
  - o Hepatic diseases
  - o Renal disease &
  - o In alcoholics
  - o Because of increased risk of lactic acidosis in all the above conditions

Starch Inhibitor:

- MOA of Acarbose & Miglitol (alpha glucosidase/ starch inhibitor):
  - o Decreases progression of impaired glucose tolerance to overt disease

Slows down and decrease digestion and absorption of polysaccharides and sucrose

- Special feature of Acarbose & Miglitol: They are mild anti-hyperglycaemics

Pioglitazone:

- Effect of Pio-glitazone (thiazo-lidine-diones) is: Acts by binding to PPAR-gamma (peroxisome proliferator activator receptors-gamma)
- Increases insulin sensitivity of tissues (reverse insulin resistance)

INSULIN

Insulin:

- $t_{1/2}$ of Insulin: 5 minutes
- Effect of Insulin on potassium: Promotes entry of potassium into the cell
- Difference between human & pork insulin: 1 amino acid

INSULIN PREPARATIONS

Rapid acting insulin:

- Insulin aspart,
- Lispro insulin &
- Insulin glusuline

Long acting insulin:

- Insulin glargine
- Insulin detemir

VI. DRUGS ACTING ON CARDIO-VASCULAR SYSTEM

ANTIHYPERTENSIVES

ACE Inhibitors:

- ACE inhibitors causes cough because of: Bradykinin
- C/I of ACE inhibitors:
  - o Bilateral renal artery stenosis (due to dilatation of efferent arterioles & fall in glomerular filtration pressure)
  - o Pregnancy (hypoplasia of organs),
  - o Phaeochromocytoma
- Act by blocking conversion of angiotensin I to angiotensin II, decreases vasopressor activity of angiotensin II and aldosterone secretion by increasing bradykinin (causes a fall in total peripheral resistance)
- Side effects include angioedema, dry cough, hyperkalemia, taste alteration, azotemia etc.
- Members include captopril, enalapril, lisinopril

DRUGS USED IN HEART FAILURE

Digoxin:

- Therapeutic level of digoxin: 0.5 to 1.4 ng/ ml
- Toxic level of digoxin: More than 2 ng/ ml
- MOA of digoxin:
  - o Inhibit Na^+/K^+ ATPase;
  - o Increases ventricular contractile force
- Route of excretion of digoxin: Kidneys
- C/I of digoxin: HOCM
- Digoxin (electrolyte abnormality) toxicity consists of:
  - o Hypokalemia (classical finding),
  - o Hypomagnesemia

Nitrates:

- Effects of nitrates on CVS physiology:
  - o Decreases preload & afterload,
  - o Decreases myocardial oxygen consumption
- S/E of nitrates:
  - o Hypotension &
  - o Reflex tachycardia
- Long acting nitrates are NOT used chronically as: Tolerance develops (due to –SH group)

VII. DRUGS ACTING ON NERVOUS SYSTEM

ANTIDEPRESSANTS

TCA:

- Amitryptiline,
- Clomipramine

Tetracyclic antidepressants (second generation):

- Maprotiline

SSRI's:

- Fluoxetine

ANTI-EPILEPTICS

Side effect (S/E) of phenytoin:

- Gum hyperplasia,
- Hydantoin syndrome
- Cerebellar atrophy
- Megaloblastic anemia
- Pseudo-Lymphoma

VIII. DRUGS ACTING ON RESPIRATORY SYSTEM

ANTI-ASTHMATICS

Theophylline (Methylxanthine):

- Theophylline metabolizing enzymes are saturable, $t^{1/2}$ is prolonged with higher doses as kinetics changes from first to zero order.
- Plasma concentrations, therefore increase disproportionately with dose
- It has a narrow margin of safety

Uses of theophylline:

- Bronchial asthma and COPD (Use in asthma has declined because of narrow margin of safety and limited efficacy).
- It is more useful in COPD
- Apnoea in premature infant

MOA of theophylline & doxophylline:

- Inhibits phospho-di-esterase 4 (PDE4)
  - o Theophylline is a subtype nonselective and weak PDE inhibitor, but PDE4 inhibition is mainly responsible for bronchodilatation.
- Release of Ca^{2+} from sarcoplasmic reticulum, especially in skeletal muscle and cardiac muscle
- Blockade of adenosine receptors

Drugs affecting metabolism of Theophylline:

- Factors decreasing theophylline levels by enhancing its metabolism primarily by inducing CYP1A2:
  - o Smoking (increase dose of theophylline by 1.6),
  - o Microsomal enzyme inducers like rifampicin and phenytoin (increase dose of theophylline by 1.5)
- Factors which increases plasma levels of theophylline by inhibiting its metabolism:
  - o Erythromycin,
  - o Ciprofloxacin,
  - o Cimetidine,
  - o Allopurinol
  - o Dose should be reduced to 2/3

Sodium cromoglycate:

- Not absorbed orally
- Administered as an aerosol through metered dose inhaler
- MOA of sodium chromoglycate/ Cromolyn sodium (used for prophylaxis):
  - o Inhibitor of mast cell degranulation (as well as other inflammatory cells) by trigger stimuli.
  - o Release of mediators of asthma like histamine, leukotrienes, PAF interleukins, etc, is restricted

Uses of Cromolyn sodium:

- Bronchial asthma (long-term prophylactic in mild-moderate asthma)
- Allergic rhinitis and allergic conjunctivitis

Montelukast:

- MOA of Montelukast:
  - o Leukotriene receptor antagonist/ LTRA
  - o It competitively antagonize $cysLT_1$ receptor mediated bronchoconstriction, airway mucus secretion, increased vascular permeability and recruitment of eosinophils.

Uses of monteleukast:

- Used in maintenance therapy of asthma (prophylactic therapy for mild-moderate asthma as alternatives to inhaled glucocorticoids)
- Modestly effective in asprin-induced asthma and exercise induced asthma

Monteleukast is NOT useful in:

- Acute attacks of asthma (they are not to be used for terminating asthma episodes)

Zileuton:

- Zileuton inhibits:
  - o 5 Lipo-oxygenase
  - o It blocks LTC_4/D_4 as well as LTB_4 synthesis
- Clinical efficacy in asthma is similar to montelukast
- Duration of action is short and it has hepatotoxic potential
- These limitations have restricted its use

Steroids in asthma:

- They are not bronchodilators
- They benefit by reducing bronchial hyperactivity, mucosal edema and suppressing inflammatory response to AG: AB (antigen: antibody) reaction

- Systemic steroid therapy is resorted to in asthma in severe chronic asthma (not controlled by bronchodilators and inhaled steroids), status asthmaticus/ acute asthma exacerbation and COPD
- S/E of inhaled steroids (Beclomethasone dipropionate, Budesonide and Fluticasone):
  - o Oropharyngeal candidiasis, hoarseness of voice, dysphonia, sore throat
  - o These can be minimized by the use of a spacer, gargling after every dose (to wash off the drug deposited on oral and pharyngeal mucosa) and prevented as well as treated by topical nystatin/ clotrimazole
- S/E of topical steroids: Glaucoma
- S/E of parenteral steroids: Posterior subcapsular cataract

IX. ANTIMICROBIAL DRUGS

ANTIBACTERIAL

Mechanism of action:

- Drugs which inhibits cross-linking (transpeptidases) & impairs cell wall synthesis:
  - o Penicillins (The beta-lactam antibiotics inhibit the transpeptidases so that cross-linking, which maintains the close knit structure of the cell wall, does not take place)
  - o Cephalosporins (all cephalosporins are bactericidal and have the same mechanism as penicillin)
  - o Vancomycin (it acts by inhibiting bacterial cell wall synthesis by binding to the terminal dipeptide 'D-ala-D-ala' sequence of peptidoglycan units),
  - o Imipenem,
  - o Aztreonam (a novel beta-lactam antibiotic in which the other ring is missing hence monobactam)
- Drugs binding to 30s ribosomal unit & inhibiting protein synthesis:
  - o Aminoglycosides,
  - o Tetracyclines

Trimethorpim/ TMP:

- MOA of trimethoprim: Inhibit nucleotide synthesis of tetra-hydro-folate by inhibiting DHFRase (DiHydro-Folate Reductase)
- Related to the antimalarial drug pyrimethamine, which selectively inhibits DHFRase
- TMP is >50,000 times more active against bacterial DHFRase than against the mammalian enzyme. Thus, human folate metabolism is not interfered at antibacterial concentrations of TMP

Cotrimoxazole:

- Individually, both sulfonamide and trimethoprim are bacteriostatic, but the combination becomes cidal against many organisms
- Ratio of sulfamethoxazole/ SMO: TMP is 5:1, because TMP enters many tissues, has a large of volume of distribution than SMO and attains lower plasma concentrations.
- DOC in p. carinii & nocardiosis: Co-trimoxazole/ CTM (pneumocystis jiroveci causes severe pneumonia in neutropenic and AIDS patients; CTM has prophylactic as well as therapeutic value, but high doses are needed)

Fluoroquinolones/ FQs:

- Block DNA topo-isomerases IV (gram positive), which nicks and separates daughter DNA strands after DNA replication
- Inhibit bacterial DNA gyrase (gram negative), which nicks double stranded DNA, introduces negative supercoils and then reseals the nicked ends.
- In place of DNA gyrase or topoismoerase IV, the mammalian cell possess an enzyme topoisomerase II (that also removes positive supercoils) which has very low affinity for FQs – hence the low toxicity to host cells.

Penicillinase-resistant (resist degradation by staphylococcal penicillinase) drugs:

- Methicillin (acid labile so must be injected; highly penicillinase resistant),
- Cloxacillin/ Dicloxacillin (Highly penicillinase and well as acid resistant; more active than methicillin against penicillinase producing staph, but not against MRSA)

Cephalosporin effective against gram negative enterobacteriacea (3rd generation):

- Parenteral:
  - o Cefoperazone (anti-pseudomonal activity),
  - o Cefotaxime
  - o Ceftriaxone
  - o Ceftazidime
  - o Ceftizoxime
- Oral:
  - o Cefixime
  - o Cefpodoxime
  - o Cefdinir
  - o Ceftibuten
  - o Ceftamet

Use of Quinupristin/ Dalfopristin (bacteriostatic):

- Gram positive cocci including MRSA, some VRSA and Vancomycin resistant enterococcus faecium (VREF)
- It inhibits bacterial protein synthesis

Imipenem:

- It is inhibited by: Dehydropeptidase I (hence given along with cilastatin)
- Imipenem is an extremely potent and broad-spectrum beta-lactam antibiotic
- Cilastatin has matched pharmacokinetics with imipenem (half –life of both is 1 hour)

Linezolid:

- Linezolid is used in: Methicillin-resistant Staphylococcus aureus (MRSA) and some VRSA, VRE etc.
- Linezolid inhibits protein synthesis
- Binds to the 23S fraction (P site) of the 50S ribosome and interfere with formation f the tRNA (f-Met)-70S initiation complex
- It is primarily bacteriostatic

Azithromycin:

- Azalide congener of erythromycin
- High activity over respiratory pathogens
- Acid-stability, rapid oral absorption (from empty stomach), larger volume of distribution
- Doesn't affect hepatic CYP3A4 enzyme
- Azithromycin is effective against:
  - o Chylamydia trachomatis (non-specific urethritis and genital infections, LGV, chlamydial pneumonia)
  - o Mycoplasma
  - o Calymmatobacter granulomatosis (donovanosis),
  - o Legionella (Legionnaire's disease)
  - o Chancroid

Vancomycin:

- A glycopeptide antibiotic
- Acts by inhibiting cell wall synthesis. It binds to the terminal dipeptide 'D-ala-D-ala' sequence of peptidoglycan units – prevents its release from the bactoprenol lipid carrier so that assembly of the units at the cell membrane and their cross linking to form the cell wall cannot take place
- S/E of vancomycin: Red man syndrome (Rapid I/V injection of vancomycin has caused chills, fever, urticaria and intense flushing – called "Red man syndrome)
- DOC for MRSA infection: Vancomycin
- Drug used for pseudo-membranous colitis (caused by C. difficile): Vancomycin (But DOC is metronidazole)

Clindamycin:

- Exhibits partial cross resistance with erythromycin
- Inhibits most gram-positive cocci
- Oral absorption is good

- Use of clindamycin is restricted to anaerobic and mixed infections, especially those involving Bact. fragilis
- MOA of clindamycin: Binds to 50s ribosomal subunit & inhibits protein subunit (similar to erythromycin)
- Drug implicated in pseudomembranous colitis: Clindamycin (one of the major problem is diarrhoea and pseudomembranous colitis due to C. difficile superinfection which is potentially fatal)

Tetracycline/ TTC:

- Primarily bacteriostatic
- Inhibit protein synthesis by binding to 30S ribosomes.
- Subsequent to such binding, attachment of aminoacyl-tRNA to the acceptor (A) site of mRNA-ribosome complex is interfered with.
- Most TTC are primarily excreted in urine by glomerular filtration; dose has to be reduced in renal failure; doxycycline is an exception to this
- Demeclocycline antagonizes ADH action and hence tried in inappropriate ADH secretion
- Complication arising due to use of outdated tetracycline/ TTC:
  - o Reversible Fanconi's syndrome (caused by degraded products – epitetracycline, anhydrotetracycline and epianhydrotetracycline which damage proximal tubules in kidney)
- S/E of tetracycline:
  - o Teratogenic,
  - o Super-infections (TTC cause more marked suppression of the resident flora;
    - – Intestinal superinfection by candida albicans is most prominent
    - – Higher doses suppress the flora more completely – greater chance of superinfection so doses on lower side of range should be used whenever possible)
  - o Tooth discoloration (TTC have chelating property).
    - – Calcium-TTC chelate gets deposited in developing teeth and bone.
    - – Given from midpregnancy to 5 months of extra-uterine life, the deciduous teeth are affected)
- S/E of doxycycline: Photo-dermatitis (but highest with Demeclocycline and low with TTC)

Chloramphenicol/ CMP:

- Primarily bacteriostatic
- CMP was highly active against Salmonella including S. typhi
- Highly chloramphenicol resistant S. typhi have emerged due to transfer of R factor by conjugation
- It crosses placenta and is secreted in bile and milk
- Primarily conjugated with glucuronic acid in the liver and little is excreted unchanged in urine
- It is most important cause of aplastic anemia, agranulocytosis & thrombocytopenia (bone marrow depression)
- MOA of chloramphenicol: Bind to 50s subunit near the acceptor (A) site and prevents peptide bond formation between the newly attached amino acid and the nascent peptide chain without interfering with the aminoacyl-tRNA attachment to the 30S ribosomes (the step blocked by TTC)

Sparfloxacin:

- Most phototoxic & longest acting quinolone: Sparfloxacin (recipients should be cautioned not to go out in the sun)
- Sparfloxacin has been discontinued in many countries including USA, but not yet in India

Sulfonamide-pyrimethamine (S/Py):

- Both components are slow acting, the combination act faster, so that it can be employed as a clinical curative, particularly for P. falciparum.
- Efficacy against P. vivax is rather low.

- By the addition of sulfonamide, development of resistance to Py is retarded
- DOC in toxoplasmosis: Sulphamethoxazole + Pyrimethamine (it is the first choice for toxopasmosis, which mainly occurs in immunocompromised patients)

Penicillin-G/ PnG:

- Narrow spectrum antibiotic
- Penicillinase is a narrow spectrum beta-lactamase which opens the beta-lactam ring and inactivates PnG
- Use has declined very much due to fear of causing anaphylaxis
- DOC in syphilis: Penicillin G (T. apllidum has not shown any resistance and PnG is the drug of choice)
- DOC in actino-mycosis: Penicillin-G (PnG is the drug of choice for rare infections like anthrax, actinomycosis, rat bite fever and those caused by Listeria monocytogenes, Pasteurella multicoda)
- Chemo-prophylactic agent for Rheumatic fever: Benzathine penicillin/ BPn (low concentrations of penicillin prevent colonization by streptococci that are indirectly responsible for rheumatic fever; BPn 1.2 MU every 4 weeks till 18 years of age or 5 years after an attack, whichever is more)

Levofloxacin:

- Oral bioavailability is nearly 100%
- Single dose is sufficient because of slower elimination and higher potency
- Indicated in community acquired pneumonia and exacerbations of chronic bronchitis.
- DOC in legionella: Azithromycin/ Levofloxacin

Ceftriaxone:

- Longer duration of action (half life: 8 hour), permitting once, or at the most twice daily dosing.
- Hypoprothrombinaemia and bleeding are the specific adverse effects
- DOC in gonorrhea: Ceftriaxone (a single dose of 250 mg I/V has proven curative in gonorrhoea)

AMINOGLYCOSIDES

MOA of aminoglycosides/ AGS:

- Inhibit translation (transport of the aminoglycoside through the bacterial cell wall and cytoplasmic membrane followed by binding to 30S ribosomes by streptomycin; other AGS bind to additional sites on 50S subunit as well as to 30S-50S interface)
- Bactericidal (this action is concentration dependent; i.e. rate of bacterial cell killing is directly related to the ratio of the peak antibiotic concentration to the MIC value. They also exert a long and concentration dependent 'post antibiotic effect')
- Distributed only extra-cellularly

S/E of aminoglycosides:

- Teratogenic (fetal ototoxicity),
- Ototoxic (most important dose and duration of treatment related adverse effect)
- Nephrotoxic (provided the drug is promptly discontinued, renal damage caused by aminoglycosides is totally reversible)
- Causes neuromuscular blockade (reduce Ach release from the motor nerve endings; Neomycin and streptomycin have higher propensity whereas tobramycin is least likely to produce this side effect; this can be partially antagonized by I/V injection of a calcium salt) (should not be used in myasthenia gravis)

Streptomycin:

- Obtained from Streptomyces griseus
- Relatively narrow antimicrobial spectrum
- Can cause vestibular disturbances
- Lowest nephrotoxicity among aminoglycosides

- Streptomycin is used in:
  - o Plague (effects rapid cure in 7-12 days; TTC have been more commonly used for mass treatment of suspected cases during an epidemic)
  - o Tularemia (effects cure in 7-10 days)

ANTI-MALARIAL

Quinine:

- DOC for cerebral malaria: Quinine
- S/E of quinine:
  - o Cinchonism: Ringing in ears, nausea, vomiting, difficulty in hearing & visual defects
  - o Hemolysis ® hemoglobinuria (black water fever)
  - o Hypoglycemia (especially in pregnancy)

Primaquine:

- Primaquine is effective for: Radical cure of plasmodium vivax
- Primaquine is ineffective against: Plasmodium falciparum
- S/E of primaquine: Hemolysis in G6PD deficients

ANTI-FUNGAL

Amphotericin B:

- Disrupts fungal cell membrane by binding to ergosterol
- The polyenes (AMB) have high affinity for ergosterol present in fungal cell membrane.
- They combine with it, get inserted into the membrane and several polyene molecule together orient themselves in such a way as to form a 'micropore'.
- MOA of amphotericin B: Forms micropores in fungal cell membrane (it has affinity for ergosterol)
- Used for systemic mycoses and intrathecally for fungal meningitis
- It binds to ergosterol and forms pores in membrane which promote leakage of electrolytes
- Side effects include shake and bake (fever/ chills), arrhythmias, I/V phlebitis (amphoterrible), nephrotoxicity
- Toxicity can be reduced by hydration and liposomal preparation
- AMB is given as I/V solution after diluting AMB powder with glucose solution
- Conventional formulation of Amphotericin B/ C-AMB intravenously, is given along with: Glucose solution (after test dose)

KCZ:

- Used for candida, blastomyces and histoplasma
- Side effects include liver dysfunction (as it inhibits cytochrome P-450) and gynecomastia
- MOA of ketoconazole: Inhibits fungal lanosterol 14-demethylase,

Impairing ergosterol (fungal steroid) synthesis

ANTI-VIRAL

Ganciclovir:

- Inhibits viral DNA polymerase
- Mutated CMV DNA polymerase may lead to development of resistance
- May cause thrombocytopenia, neutropenia and leukopenia
- Antiviral more active against CMV: Ganciclovir

ANTI-HIV

NRTI group:

- They inhibit reverse transcriptase enzyme thus preventing incorporation of viral genome into host DNA
- Members include Zidovudine, Zalcitabine, Lamivudine, Abacavir, Didanosine and Stavudine

Abacavir:

- Belongs to Nucleoside reverse transcriptase inhibitor;
- Guanosine analogue

NNRTIs group:

- Same as that of NRTI group
- Members include Nevirapine, Etravirine, Delaviridine and Efavirenz
- Nevirapine & Efavirenz belongs to: Non-nucleoside reverse transcriptase inhibitor

Protease inhibitor group:

- They block protease in progeny virions thus inhibiting assembly of new virus
- Members include Ritonavir, Nelfinavir, Saquinavir, Indinavir, Amprenavir
- Saquinavir & Nelfinavir belongs to: Protease inhibitor

S/E of Zidovudine:

- Myelosuppression,
- Megaloblastic anemia (macrocytosis)
- Neutropenia,
- Myopathy (skeletal and cardiac)

S/E of didanosine:

- Pancreatitis,
- Peripheral neuropathy,
- Hyperuricemia,
- Seizures etc.

ANTI-TUBERCULAR

INH:

- MOA of Isoniazid/ INH: Inhibits mycolic acid cell wall synthesis via oxygen-dependent pathways
- Anti-TB drug showing maximum resistance in India: INH
- Special feature about activity of INH:
  - o Bacterio-static against resting bacilli
  - o Bacterio-cidal against rapidly multi-plying organism
  - o (both intra-cellularly & extra-cellularly present organism)
- Treatment of INH related peripheral neuritis:
  - o 100 mg of pyridoxine daily for treatment and
  - o 10 mg/ day for prophylaxis (orally)
- S/E of INH:
  - o Peripheral neuritis (common in slow acetylator)
  - o Hepatotoxicity (common in elderly & alcoholics; rare in children
  - o Seizures (neurotoxicity)
  - o Optic neuritis
  - o Hemolysis in G-6-PD deficients
  - o SLE like syndrome

S/E of rifampicin:

- Respiratory syndrome
- Abdominal syndrome
- Flu like syndrome
- Cutaneous syndrome
- Hepatotoxicity
- Orange coloured urine and sweat
- P-450 drug interactions (microsomal enzyme inducer) etc.

Pyrazinamide:

- Special features of pyrazinamide:
  - o Levels in CSF are high (good penetration in CSF)
  - o Bacteriocidal to organism lying within caseous granuloma (acidic pH) and slowly dividing intracellular bacteria
- MOA of pyrazinamide:
  - o Similar to INH (inhibition of mycolic acid cell wall synthesis) but by interacting with a different fatty acid synthase encoding gene (but intracellular action)
  - o More active at pH <6
- Side effects (3H):
  - o Hepatotoxicity (less in Indians)
  - o Hyperuricemia
  - o Hyperglycemia

S/E of ethambutol:

- Retrobulbar optic neuritis
- Color vision disturbance (red-green)
- Never given to children's less than 5 years of age as they can't complain about visual problems.

ANTI-LEPROTIC

Rifampicin:

- Most rapidly acting drug against leprosy bacillus: Rifampicin
- Most potent drug against leprosy bacillus: Rifampicin

Dapsone:

- DOC for leprosy: Dapsone
- S/E of dapsone: Hemolysis in G6PD deficient

S/E of clofazimine:

- Reddish black discoloration of skin,
- Acneform eruptions

ANTI-PARASITIC DRUSG

SSG:

- Has been the first line drug for visceral leishmaniasis/ VL in most parts of the world achieving >90% cure rate, but is no longer effective in India and
- Nepal because of extensive resistance.
- Over 60% cases in Bihar are unresponsiveness to SSG
- DOC in kala-azar: Sodium stibogluconate (SSG is administered by deep I/M injection into buttocks or by slow I/V injection daily or on alternate days)

Miltefosine:

- Was approved in 2002 as the first orally active drug for kala-azar
- Due to spread of SSG resistance in Bihar and neighbouring areas, NVBDCP is now using mitefosine as the 1st line treatment of VL in India.
- A 4 week course has achieved >95% cure rate in India
- Oral drug for kala-azar: Miltefosine (it is rapidly absorbed after oral medication, and widely distributed in the body)

MNZ:

- It is bactericidal
- It forms toxic metabolites in the bacterial cell damaging DNA
- Used as antiprotozoal drug (amoebiasis, giardiasis, bacterial vaginosis) and triple therapy for H. pylori
- Can lead to Disulfiram-like reaction, metallic taste
- DOC for dracunculiasis: Metronidazole/ MNZ

X. ANTI-NEOPLASTIC DRUGS

CANCER CHEMOTHERAPY

Uses of cetumixab:

- Acts against epidermal growth factor receptor (EGFR) positive colo-rectal cancer (as a single agent)
- Advanced/ metastatic squamous Ca of head & neck region

IMMUNOSUPPRESANTS

Cyclosporin:

- MOA of cyclosporin (immunosuppressant): It profoundly & selectively inhibits T lymphocyte proliferation, IL-2 & other cytokine production
- Lymphocytes are arrested in G0/ G1 phase
- Cyclosporin acts on: CD4+ T-cells

Tacrolimus:

- MOA of Tacrolimus: Same as cyclosporin; Acts mainly on T-cells
- Use of tacrolimus: Organ transplantation

Bromocriptine:

- Bromocriptine inhibits: Prolactin secretion
- Bromocriptine is indicated in:
  - o Galactorrhea (due to hyperprolactinoma);
  - o Infertility (due to hyperprolactinoma);
  - o In acromegaly,
  - o Idiopathic/ post-encephalitic parkinsonism (along with levo-dopa/ carbidopa)

Octreotide is used in:

- Varices/ esophageal bleeding;
- May be used in AIDS patients with secretory diarrhea (who have failed to respond to antimicrobial or antimotility agents)

CHAPTER 6

MICROBIOLOGY & PARASITOLOGY

I. GENERAL MICROBIOLOGY

BASICS

Prokaryotes:

- In prokaryotes, nuclear membrane is: Absent.
- In prokaryotes, cellular organelles are: Absent
- They do not have organelles except ribsomes (70s)
- They contain single circular molecule of loosely organized DNA lacking a
- nuclear membrane and mitotic apparatus

Dark ground microscopy:

- Detection of flagella (and hence motility)
- Visualization of live thin organism like spirochete

Major encapsulated organism:

- Streptococcus
- Klebsiella
- H. influenza
- Pseudomonas
- Neisseria
- Cryptococcus
- Capsules are detected by: Quellung reaction/ Indian ink

Conjugation (horizontal gene transfer):

- Donor is determined by specific conjugate plasmids called fertility plasmids (F+) or sex plasmids
- Multiple drug resistance

EXOTOXIN & ENDOTOXIN

Exotoxin & Endotoxin:

- Mostly secreted by gram positive bacteria: Exotoxin
- Endotoxin is secreted only by gram negative bacteria (component of cell wall)
- Highly toxic: Exotoxin
- Endotoxin have low toxicity
- Highly antigenic: Exotoxin (induces synthesis of protective antibody in host called antitoxin)
- Endotoxin is poorly antigenic
- Toxoids are used as vaccines: Exotoxin
- No toxoids, so no vaccines from endotoxin

Exotoxin:

- Polypeptides (endotoxin are lipopolys-accharide)
- Delicate/ heat labile (endotoxin are heat resistant)

II. BACTERIOLOGY

STAPHYLOCCCUS AURUES

Staph aureus:

- Gram +
- Catalase +
- Coagulase +
- Causes folliculitis, bullous impetigo, osteomyelitis, surgical wound infections
- Food poisoning results due to: Preformed enterotoxin

- Incubation period of staph. aureus food poisoning: Less than 6 hours
- Staphy. aureus food poisoning is seen after ingestion of: Dairy products

Staph epidermidis:

- Gram +
- Catalase +
- Coagulase –
- Causes I/V cannula & prosthesis related infections

Toxins of Staph:

- Epidermolytic toxin (exfoliative toxin): SSS
- Enterotoxin
- Toxic shock syndrome toxin

STREPTOCOCCI

Beta hemolytic streptococci:

- A: S. Pyogenes (Bacitracin sensitive, CAMP -)
- B: S. Agalactaciae (Bacitracin resistant, CAMP +)
- D: S. fecalis & S. bovis

Classification based on hemolysis:

- Alpha: Viridans group
- Beta: Most of the pathogenic (Lancefield classification based on carbohydrate antigen)
- Gamma: Enterococci

Disease caused by Streptococcus pyogenes (GABHS):

- Pharyngitis/ sore throat
- Scarlet fever
- Impetigo
- Erysipelas
- Cellulitis
- Toxic Shock Syndrome (2nd MC)

PNEUMOCOCCUS

Pneumococcus:

- Alpha hemolytic
- Bile soluble, Optochin sensitive
- Quellung reaction (capsular polysaccharide antigen)
- C-reactive protein (precipitates C-carbohydrate antigen)
- MC cause of lobar pneumonia & pyogenic meningitis
- Most virulent type of pneumococcus: Type C
- Appearance of colonies: Draughtsman colonies
- Gross appearance of pneumococcus: Lanceolate, Flame shaped diplococcus

NEISSERIA

Condition caused by N. gonorrhoeae:

- Ophthalmia neonatorum (babies born to infected mother)
- Male: Urethritis (does not involve testis)
- Female: Cervicitis
- Complications:
  - o Deep gonococcal infections
  - o Endocarditis (rarely),
  - o Commonly purulent arthritis
- Special feature:
  - o Intra-cytoplasmic,
  - o Gram negative,
  - o Non-capsulated,
  - o Kidney shaped,
  - o Ferments glucose

N. meningitidis:

- Capsulated
- Lens shaped, half-moon shaped (adjacent surfaces flat)
- Ferments glucose and maltose
- Waterhouse-Friderichsen syndrome (fulminant meningococcemia)
- Thayer Martin media (culture media)

CORYNEBACTERIUM DIPHTHERIAE

C. diphtheriae:

- Club-shaped, irregularly stained gram-positive pleomorphic rod

- Chinese letter/ cuneiform arrangement (V-L shaped in smear)

Culture media for C. diphtheriae:

- Loeffler's serum slope
  - o Enriched media
  - o Growth can be detected as early as 6-8 hours
  - o Best medium for metachromatic granules production
- Hoyle's potassium Tellurite media/ PTA:
  - o Selective media
  - o C. diphtheriae reduces tellurite to metallic tellurium producing black colour

Babes Ernest granules/ Volutin granules/ Metachromatic granules/ Polar bodies:

- Present at the ends/ poles of bacilli
- Storage granules of the organism, composed of polymetaphosphates

B. ANTHRACIS

B. anthracis:

- Gram +ve, large rectangular rods arranged in chains, non-motile and capsulated, non-bulging oval spores
- It was the first pathogenic bacterium seen under microscope
- Anthrax vaccine was the 1st live attenuated bacterial vaccine prepared

Anthrax:

- Zoonosis,
- Human beings acquire infection by cutaneous mode (by spores entering through abraded skin), inhalation of spores, ingestion of carcasses of animals dying of anthrax containing spores
- McFadyean's reaction positive
- Polypeptide capsule can be demonstrated by staining with Gurr's polychrome methylene blue stain for 30 seconds.
- Capsule appears as amorphous purple material surrounding blue bacilli.

Pulmonary anthrax:

- Wool sorters disease (as it is seen in workers of wool factory, acquire infection by inhalation of dust from infected wool)
- It is rare but fatal

Cutaneous anthrax/ Hide porter's disease:

- Painless malignant pustule (charbon)
- However, it is a non-malignant condition

CLOSTRIDIA

C. difficile:

- Obligate anaerobic, gram-positive, spore forming bacillus.
- It was so named due to unusual difficulties involved in the isolation of C. difficile
- Clostridium difficile causes:
  - o Pseudomembranous colitis (particularly after antibiotic therapy)
  - o Prolonged antimicorbial use results in disruption of the normal colonic flora, which enhances the susceptibility to C. difficile infection
  - o Ceftriaxone, clindamycin, ampicillin and ciprofloxacin are implicated

C. perfringenes/ C. welchii:

- Commensal in the large intestine of human beings
- Capsulated, non-motile, gram-positive bacillus
- Bears sub-terminal bulging spores
- Clostridium perfringenes causes:
  - o Gas gangrene/ myonecrosis,
  - o Necrotizing enterocolitis,
  - o Food poisoning,
  - o Enteritis necroticans (gas gangrene of the bowel)

Tetanus:

- Tetanus bacilli enter through injury (superficial abrasions, punctured wounds, road traffic accidents), surgery done without proper asepsis, neonates (following abortion/ delivery)
- IP (Incubation period): 6-10 days
- Shorter the IP, graver is the prognosis.

- Muscles of the face and jaw are often affected first (due to shorter distances for the toxin to reach the presynaptic terminals)
- First symptom – increase in the masseter tone leading to trismus or lock jaw
- Risus sardonicus (sustained spasm of the facial muscles)
- Opisthotonus (generalised spastic contraction of the extensor muscles)

C. tetani:

- Obligate anaerobic, gram-positive bacillus with terminal round spore (drum stick appearance)
- Tetanospasmin prevents the presynaptic release of inhibitory neurotransmitters glycine and GABA, which leads to spastic muscle contraction
- Arrangement of spores of C. tetani: Drum stick appearance; round & terminal spores
- Motility of C. tetani: Motile with swarming tendency
- Culture on Blood agar with polymyxin B – C. tetani produces characteristic swarming growth
- Clostridium tetani causes: Tetanus

C. botulinum:

- Anaerobic, gram-positive bacillus with subterminal spore
- Effect of toxin of Clostridium botulinum:
  - o Blocks release of acetylcholine at neuro-muscular junction;
  - o Botulinum toxin binds to acetylcholine receptors on the nerve terminals at neuromuscular junction, which results in blockage of release of the acetylcholine, leading to flaccid paralysis

E. COLI

Enterotoxigenic E. Coli:

- MC cause for traveler's diarrhea: ETEC/ Enterogenic E. coli
- MC cause of traveler's diarrhea in 25-75% of cases
- Causes acute watery diarrhea in infants and adults

Enterohemorrhagic E. coli/ EHEC:

- EHEC secretes a verocytotoxin/ shiga-like toxin
- Shiga-like toxin causes capillary micro-angiopathy
- Most of the cases of hemolytic uremic syndrome (HUS) are caused by: EHEC/ Enterohemorrhagic E. coli
- Causes hemorrhagic colitis and HUS

Enteropathogenic E. coli/ EPEC:

- Causes infantile diarrhea (outbreaks)
- Important cause of infant diarrhea: EPEC/ Enteropathogenic E. coli
- Nontoxigenic and noninvasive

YERSINIA PESTIS

Yersinia pestis:

- Gram-negative oval coccobacillus, often shows bipolar staining (ends of the bacilli stain darker than the central part) and pleomorphism (variable size and shapes) in older cultures.
- Non-motile and capsulated
- Pattern of growth:
  - o Stalactite growth
  - o Culture on nutrient broth with oil or ghee floated on top-characteristic stalactite-like growth occurs hanging down from the undersurface of the oil.

Plague:

- MC form of plague: Bubonic plague
- Transmitted by the bite of an infected rat flea
- IP: 2-7 days
- Buboes:
  - o Regional lymph nodes appear as tense, tender swellings
  - o MC in inguinal region

...lla pertusis:

- Highly fastidious
- Very small
- Strict aerobe
- Gram-negative coccobacillus
- Grows best at 35-37 degree C
- Media used: Bordet gengou medium
  - o Bordet-Gengou glycerine-potato-blood agar was a traditional medium used before

Whooping cough:

- IP of whooping cough: 7-10 days
- Clinical course of whooping cough/ pertusis/ 100 days fever passes through 3 stages:
  - o Catarrhal stage
  - o Paroxysmal stage
  - o Convalescent stage

BRUCELLA

Brucella causes:

- Malta fever/ Undulant fever/ Mediterranean fever
- Fever has a typical remittent course, i.e. in between febrile periods (which lasts for weeks), there will be afebrile periods.

Tests for antibody detection in milk in animal brucellosis:

- Rose bengal card test,
- Whey agglutination test
- Milk ring test
  - o In milk ring test, pooled milk is mixed with a drop of the stained brucella antigen in a narrow test tube and incubated at 70 degree C for 40-50 minutes
  - o If antibodies are present in the milk, bacilli are agglutinated and rise to form a blue ring at the top, leaving the milk unstained
  - o If antibodies are absent, no coloured ring is formed and the milk remains uniformly blue

TREPONEMA PALLADIUM

Treponema pallidum:

- Extremely thin bacilli and delicate with tapering ends
- Flexible, spirally coiled
- Actively motile (corkscrew motility)
- 3-4 Endoflagellum provides motility
- Cannot be visualized by light microscope
- Specific/ Treponemal test for T. pallidum (specific antibodies are detected by using T. pallidum antigens):
  - o FTA-ABS (Fluorescent treponemal antibody absorption test)
  - o TPI (Treponema pallidum immobilization test)
  - o TPA (T. pallidum agglutination test)
  - o TPHA (T. pallidum hemagglutination test)

FTA-ABS:

- Uses killed T. pallidum
- Highly sensitive and specific in all the stages of syphilis
- First serological test to be positive after infection
- IgM-FTA-ABS test is another modification used for congenital syphilis.
- It detects IgM antibodies in fetal serum

VDRL:

- A type of non-treponemal test/ non-specific test/ standard tests
- It is most widely used, simple and rapid serological test
- It is preferred for field studies and antenatal screening
- VDRL is positive in: Syphilis
- Secondary syphilis is characterized by skin and mucous membranes involvement (skin rashes, condyloma lata, mucosal patches)
- VDRL (Veneral disease research laboratory) is a type of: Slide flocculation test

- Other slide flocculation tests:
  - o RPR (Rapid plasma reagin),
  - o USR (Unheated serum reagin),
  - o TRUST (Toluidine red unheated serum test)

OTHER BACTERIA

Proteus:

- Peritrichate flagella
- Urease positive (urease breaks down urea to form ammonia that damages renal epithelium and makes the urine alkaline)
- Dienes phenomenon:
  - o When two strains of Proteus are inoculated at different areas on culture plate:
  - – If swarming of two strains merge completely, and remain separated by a narrow line of demarcation – indicates two strains are different
  - – If swarming of two strains merge completely without any line of demarcation – indicates two strains are identical
- Effect of urease, produced by proteus:
  - o Urease hydrolyzes urea to ammonia, which results in alkalinization of urine
  - o Hence high prevalence of UTI in long-term catheterized individuals
- Alkaline urine predisposes to the deposition of phosphate, which leads to the formation of struvite calculi

Shigella:

- Most important agent of bacillary dysentery
- Nonmotile and not fermenting most sugars except mannitol
- Based on somatic O polysaccharide antigen, shigella is divided into 4 groups
  - o Group A: S. dysenteriae
  - o Group B: S. flexneri
  - o Group C: S. boydii
  - o Group D: S. sonnei
- Division of shigella is done on the basis of: Mannitol fermentation
- All species of shigella ferment mannitol except S. dysenteriae, Newcastle biotype of S. flexneri serotype-6 and rabaulensis biotype of S. flexneri serotype-4a
- Most virulent type is:
  - o S. Dysentriae (group A): It does not ferment mannitol, in contrast to other species of Shigella, which are mannitol fermenters.
- Best test for S. dysentriae: Stool culture
  - o Fresh stool is collected
  - o To inhibit the commensals, fecal specimen is inoculated simultaneously into enrichment broth (Selenite F broth) and selective media (MacConkey agar)

Salmonella:

- Motile
- Non-sporing
- Non-capsulated
- Gram-negative bacilli
- Peritrichous flagella except S. Gallinarum and S. Pullorum
- ICUT test:
  - o Indole test (-ve),
  - o Citrate test (+ve except S. typhi and S. paratyphi A),
  - o Urease test (-ve) &
  - o Triple sugar iron test
- Factor needed for growth: Tryptophan
- Most immunogenic antigen: H. Antigen
  - o Flagellar antigen (made up of flagellin)
  - o Confers motility
  - o Appears late and disappears late
  - o Indicates convalescent stage
- Carriers are detected by: Vi antigen
  - o Capsular antigen covering the O antigen
  - o Vi antigen stands for virulence
  - o Vi antigen is not helpful in diagnosis (so not employed in Widal test)
  - o Vi antibody, if persists indicates the development of the carrier state

Vibrio cholerae:

- Curved
- Gram-negative bacilli

- Actively motile by means of single polar flagellum
- Serogroup:
  - o O1,
  - o NAG vibrios (non-agglutinable),
  - o O139,
  - o Non O1/ O139 serogroup
- Biotyping:

Serogroup O1 has 2 biotypes:

- o Classical &
- o El Tor (responsible for all outbreaks of cholera)
- Isolation of V. cholerae was done by: Koch
- Robert Koch isolated the organism in 1886, and names it as Komma bacillus (due to its characteristic curved or comma-shaped appearance)
- Motility of V. cholerae:
  - o Darting motility
  - o Hanging drop method shows actively motile bacilli, with frequently changing direction, described as darting/ shooting star/ swarming gnats motility (dart means a small, slender, pointed missile which shows sudden, rapid movement when thrown at a target)
- Special features of vibrio cholerae:
  - o Non-halophilic
  - o Cant grow in media with a concentration of NaCl more than 7%
  - o NaCl (0.5-1%) stimulates the growth, however, high concentrations of NaCl are inhibitory
- Transported in alkaline medium (8.2):
  - o VR medium
  - o Cary-Blair medium

Pseudomonas:

- Oxidase-positive
- Pigment producing
- Non-fermenting
- Gram-negative bacilli
- Major pathogen among the hospitalized patients and in patients with cystic fibrosis
- It causes:
  - o VAP (ventilator associated pneumonia)
  - o Malignant otitis externa
- Pyoverdin/ Fluorescin (greenish yellow) is: One of the pigment produced by P. aeruginosa
- Pseudomonas produces a number of pigments which diffuse freely into the surroundings
  - o Pyocyanin: Blue green pigment (produced only by P. aeruginosa)
  - o Pyorubin: Red color
  - o Pyomelanin: Brown black color

Hemophilus:

- Oxidase positive,
- Capsulated
- Pleomorphic
- Gram-negative bacilli that require special growth factors present in blood, such as factor X and V (Haemo means blood, philus means loving)
- Factors required for growth:
  - o Factor V & X
  - o Hemophilus require these 2 accessory growth factors present in blood
- Appearance on H. ducreyi on culture: School of fish
  - o On direct microscopy, H. ducreyi is a pleomorphic gram-negative coccobacillus; occurs in groups or in parallel chains.
  - o They frequently take bipolar staining.
  - o This arrangement has been described as school of fish/ rail road track arrangement.

Mycobacterium tuberculosis:

- Non-motile,
- Non-sporing
- Non-capsulated
- Weakly gram-positive
- Straight or slightly curved rod-shaped bacteria
- Which are obligate aerobes (or microaerophilic).

- They sometimes show branching filamentous forms resembling fungal mycelium (myces means fungus)
- M. bacilli was discovered by: Robert Koch
  - o Robert Koch (1882) isolated the tubercle bacillus and proved its causative role in tuberculosis as it satisfies the Koch's postulates
- Factor responsible for acid fastness: Mycolic acid & cell wall
  - o Mycolic acid layer is the principal constituent, made up of long chain fatty acids attached to arabinogalactam.
  - o It confers very low permeability to the cell wall and is responsible for acid fastness and also reduces the entry of most antibiotics
- Stain used for rapid diagnosis (screening) of M. bacilli: Auramine phenol stain
  - o Auramine phenol technique is a fluorescent technique, uses auramine phenol as primary stain, acid alcohol as decolorizer and potassium permanganate as counter stain
  - o The bacilli appear bright brilliant green against dark background
- Factor which promotes virulence: Cord factor
- Special feature (which differentiates M. tb from M. bovis): Production of niacin
  - o Niacin test is positive for M. tuberculosis and rarely for few strains of M. simiae and M. cheloneii.
  - o However this is negative for M. bovis

Mycobacterium leprae:

- Strict aerobe and
- Obligately intracellular bacilli
- Less acid fast as compared to tubercle bacilli
- Not cultivable either in artificial culture media or in tissue culture (so doesn't follow Koch's postulates)
- Generation time of M. leprae: 12-13 days
  - o Long generation time of 12-13 days as compared to 14 hours in tubercle bacillus and about 20 minutes for coliform bacilli
- M. leprae can be maintained in:
  - o Foot pad of mice (kept at low temperature, 20 degree C)
  - o Lepra bacilli can also be maintained in animals, such as nine banded armadillo (Dasypus novemcinctus)
- M. leprae spreads by:
  - o Prolonged contact with patients, who discharged bacilli in nasal secretions (nasal droplet infection)
    - – A sneeze from an untreated lepromatous leprosy patient may contain >10^{10} lepra bacilli
  - o Contact transmission (skin):
    - – Direct contact from person to person
    - – Indirect contact with infected soil, fomites such as clothes and linens
- Virchows Lepra cells are present in: Macrophages
  - o AFB are seen either singly or in groups (cigar like bundles), bound together by lipid-like substance, the glia to form globi.
  - o The globi are present inside the foamy macrophages called Virchow's lepra cells or foamy cells

Borrelia:

- Poorly gram-stained (other spirochaetes do not take Gram stain)
- 7-11 endoflagellum
- Better viewed under dark ground microscope or by silver impregnation staining
- Lymes disease/ erythema migrans is caused by: B. Burgdorferi
- Isolation of B. burgdorferi can be done in special medium called BSK medium (Barbour-Stoenner-Kelly)
- Relapsing fever is caused by: B. Recurrentis
  - o Most reliable serological method for B. recurrentis is GlpQ (Glycerophosphodiester phosphodiesterase) assay

Leptospira interrogans:

- Tightly and regularly coiled, with characteristic hooked ends (interrogans resembling interrogation/ questions marks)

- Single endoflagellum
- Spinning and translational movements
- Cannot be seen under light microscope (lepto means fine/ thin)
- Leptospirosis is associated with:
  - o Rat,
  - o Rice,
  - o Rain
  - o The three most important epidemiological determinants for leptospirosis include exposure to rodents, rainfall and rice fields (3R's)

Mycoplasma:

- Also known as eaton agent,
- Prokaryotes, that are bounded by cell membrane &
- As they lack cell wall, they show:
  - o Cellular pleomorphism &
  - o Resistance to cell wall active antimicrobial agents (penicillins & cephalosporins)
- Appearance of colonies: Fried eggs colonies

Actinomycetes:

- Gram positive,
- Growth usually results in formation of clumps (grains/ sulfur granules)

Listeria:

- Genus received its current name, after the British pioneer of sterile urgery Joseph Lister, in 1940
- Gram positive,
- Rod-shaped
- Facultatively anaerobic
- Tumbling motility
- Test used: Anton's test
- Drug of choice for listerial meningitis: Ampicillin + Gentamicin

H. pylori:

- Gram negative,
- Spiral, flagellate bacillus,
- Produces urease
  - o Urease protects it from acid by catalyzing conversion of urea to ammonia (buffer)
- Route of transmission of H. pylori: Man to man
  - o Faeco-orally,
  - o Oro-gastric route
- MC cause of peptic ulcer

Rickettsia:

- Non-motile
- Gram-negative
- Nonspore forming
- Highly pleomorphic bacteria
- Rickettsial pox is caused by (vector: ticks): R. akari
- Q fever is caused by (only rickettsia NOT transmitted to humans by an arthropod): Coxialla burnetti

Chlamydia:

- Gram negative
- Obligate intracellular bacteria, (can grow inside a cell only)
- 2 forms:
  - o Extracellular Elementary body is metabolically inert
  - o Initial/ reticulate body which divides to form daughter elementary bodies seen as inclusion bodies (Halberstaedter-Prowazek bodies)
- Cytoplasmic inclusion bodies by Giemsa stain
- C. Psittaci is acquired by inhalation of pigeon feces
- C. Trachomatis is acquired by sexual contact or vertically at birth
  - o Serotypes A-C causes trachoma
  - o Serotypes D-K causes genitourinary infections
  - o Serotype L1-L3 causes Lymphogranuloma venerum/ LGV

III. VIROLOGY

Prions:

- Protein molecules, that can spread from cell to cell & effect changes in the structure of their normal counterparts (cellular proteins)

- o Creutzfeldt-Jakob disease,
- o Kuru,
- o Gerstmann-Straussler disease,
- o Mad cow disease,
- o Fatal familial insomnia

Viruses belonging to DNA group:

- Herpes viruses
- Hepadna viruses (Hepatitis B virus)
- Adenovirus
- Parvovirus
- Papillomavirus
- Polyomavirus (JC virus)
- Poxvirus (Smallpox, Molluscum contagiosum)

Viruses belonging to RNA group:

- Picornavirus (Poliovirus)
- Calicivirus (Hepatitis E virus)
- Reovirus (Roatvirus)
- Flavivirus (HCV, Yellow fever)
- Togavirus (Rubella)
- Retrovirus (HIV)
- Coronavirus
- Orthomyxovirus (Influenza virus)
- Paramyxovirus (Parainfluenza virus)
- Rhabdovirus (Rabies virus)
- Filovirus (Ebola virus)
- Arenavirus
- Bunyavirus
- Deltavirus (Hepatitis D virus)

Viruses belonging to herpes group:

- HSV-1 (Hereps labialis, Encephalitis)
- HSV-2 (Genital infections)
- Varicella zoster (Chickenpox, Shingles/ Herpes zoster)
- EBV (Infectious mononucleosis, Burkitt's lymphoma, Nasopharyngeal carcinoma, Oral hairy leukoplakia)
- CMV (Infection in AIDS)
- HHV-8 (Kaposi's sarcoma)

Facts related to herpes group viruses:

- MC cause of sporadic viral encephalitis: HSV
- Varicella zoster (HHV-3) virus remains dormant in: Sensory ganglion
- HSV lies dormant in trigeminal ganglion
- More than 50% of renal transplants with fever, 1-4 months after transplantation have: CMV infection (HHV-5)

Polio:

- Polio virus (inside body) spreads by:
  - o Hematogenous route,
  - o Neural route
- MC manifestation of polio is: Subclinical infection (90%)
- Death in polio is mostly due to: Respiratory paralysis

Influenza virus:

- Antigenic drift (minor change): Small mutations in H & N
- Antigenic shift (major change)
- Bird flu virus is also known as: Avian flu influenza virus/ H5N1
- Swine flu (2009 outbreak) was due to: H1N1

Measles:

- Measles virus belongs to: Paramyxovirus
- Infectivity period of measles:
  - o 4 days before rash,
  - o 5 days after rash appearance
- A rare, late neurological complication: SSPE (subacute sclerosing panencephalitis)

Mumps:

- MC complication of mumps in post-pubertal males: Orchitis
- Special feature of mumps: One attacks gives lifelong immunity

Congenital rubella triad:

- Cataract,
- Deafness,
- Heart diseases (patent ductus arteriosus)

Rabies:

- Rabies virus is: Enveloped virus with ss RNA
- Negri bodies are pathognomic of: Rabies encephalitis

- They are present: Inside nerve cells
- For ante-mortem diagnosis: Immunofluorescence

Hepatitis:

- Special feature of hepatitis A virus (previously known as enterovirus 72): No chronic course
- Hepatitis B virus contains which enzyme: DNA dependent DNA polymerase, (compare with HIV)
- Dane particle is: HBV
- HBV strain in India:
  - Ayw
  - Adr
- Maximum perinatal transmission risk for which hepatitis virus: HBV
- Serological marker of acute hepatitis B infection:
  - HBsAg
  - Core antibody (IgM anti-HBcAg)
- Epidemiological marker of Hepatitis B infection: HBsAg
- Indicator of high infectivity of hepatitis B infection:
  - HBeAg
  - HBV-DNA (indicator of intrahepatic viral replication)
- HCV belongs to which group: Flaviviridae
- MC cause of post-transfusion hepatitis: HCV
- HEV is transmitted: Enterically/ Faeco-orally
- Highest mortality in pregnancy with hepatitis is with: HEV
- Hepatitis viruses spreading by feco-oral route are:
  - HAV
  - HEV

HIV:

- HIV consists of:
  - 2 copies of ss RNA,
  - RNA dependent DNA polymerase [compare with HBV],
  - Integrase
  - Protease
- Seroconversion takes: 2-6 weeks
- Chances of transmission with accidental needle prick: 0.3%
- Retroviral sequence in host cell: RNA-DNA-RNA
- p24 antigen (used for early diagnosis) disappears after: 6-8 weeks of HIV infection
- CD4: CD8 ratio is: Reversed in HIV infection
- Window period: Time period between, infection to appearance of antibodies in serum
- During window period, ELISA & western blot are: Negative
- MC cause of diarrhea in AIDS: Cryptosporodiosis (NOT cryptococcus)
- MC cause of meningitis in AIDS: Cryptococcus
- MC cause of oral ulcer in AIDS: Candida
- MC cause of TB in AIDS in tropical countries: Mycobacterium TB
- MC opportunistic infection in AIDS in India is: TB

Rota-virus:

- Double stranded RNA virus
- Non cultivable (does not grow in cell cultures),
- Detected by antigen in stools
- MC cause of infantile diarrhea: Rota-virus

HPV:

- HPV with high oncogenic potential: HPV16, 18
- HPV causes warts, cervical intraepithelial neoplasia & cervical cancer

IV. MYCOLOGY

General facts:

- Fungi which are, spherical in tissue, but grow like molds, when cultures at room temperature are k/a: Dimorphic fungi
- Fungal cell membrane is stained by:
  - PAS,
  - Methanamine silver
- Fungi without sexual stage: Fungi imperfection

- Culture media for fungi: Saboubard's dextrose agar/ SDA
- Non-culturable fungus: Rhinosporodium

Candida:

- MC fungal infection in neutropenic patients: Candidiasis
- Reynolds Braude phenomenon is shown by: Candida
- Thrush is caused by: Candida (thrush is also k/a oral candidiasis)

Dermatophytes infect:

- Skin
- Nail
- Hair

Cryptococcus:

- Cryptococcus has predilection for: Brain
- India ink (microscopy) wet mount is used for diagnosis of: Cryptococcus capsule
- MC cause of acute meningitis in AIDS: Cryptococcus

Aspergillus:

- Hyphae in Aspergillus fumigates: Branching hyphae/ Septate
- Portal of entry of Aspergillus fumigates: Lungs (can colonize the damaged bronchial tree, pulmonary cysts, cavities of patients with underlying lung tissue)

V. PARASITOLOGY

NEMATODES/ ROUNDOWRM & HOOKWORM

Ascaris lumbricoides/ Giant roundworm:

- Eggs are visible in feces
- Bowel obstruction
- Iron deficiency

Wucheria bancrofti:

- Causes lymphatic filariasis by blocking lymphatic vessels
- Treated by DEC (DiEthylCarbamazine)

Loa Loa:

- Worm can be seen crawling in eye (conjunctiva)
- Causes Calabar swelling

Onchocerca volvulus:

- Causes river blindness
- Transmitted by female blackflies

Strongyloides stercoralis, Ancylostoma duodenale, Necator americanus (Hookworm):

- Larvae in soil penetrate the skin
- Iron deficiency anemia
- Cutaneous larva migrans

Toxocara canis:

- Visceral larva migrans
- Causes granulomas

Enterobius vermicularis/ Pinworm:

- Food contaminated with eggs
- Causes anal pruritus

Dracunculus medinensis/ Guinea worm:

- Largest nematode
- Causes inflammation & ulceration of skin

CESTODES/ TAPEWORMS

Echinocoocus granulosus/ Dog tapeworm:

- Ingestion of eggs (in dog feces) can result in cyst in liver (Hydatid cyst)

Taenia solium/ Pork tapeworm:

- Causes cysticercosis & neurocysticercosis
- Ingestion of larvae encysted in undercooked pork
- Definitive host: Humans
- Intermediate host: Pig

TREMATODES

Schistosoma Japonicum:

- Host: Snails
- Causes: Urinary bladder carcinoma, hematuria

MICROFILARIA

Microscopy of microfilaria:

- Microfilariae bancrofti: Tail tip free from nuclei
- Micrfilariae malayi: Nuclei till tail tip

PROTOZOA

Entamoeba histolytica:

- Amoebic dysentery (bloody diarrhoea)
- Extra-intestinal: Amoebic liver abscess

Giardia lamblia/ intestinalis:

- Foul smelling, non-bloody diarrhoea
- Treated by metronidazole

Trichomonas vaginalis:

- Trichominiasis presents with green colored, foul smelling discharge
- Motile trophozoites can be seen on wet mount

Leishmania donovani:

- Causes kala-azar/ visceral leishmaniasis
- Transmitted by sand-fly

Cryptosporodium:

- Causes severe diarrhoea in AIDS

Naegleria fowleri:

- Causes rapidly fatal meningo-encephalitis

Trypanosoma cruzi:

- Causes Chagas disease in South America
- Transmitted by Reduvid bug

Trypanosoma brucei:

- Causes African sleepin sickness
- Transmitted by TseTse fly

PLASMODIA

4 types of plasmodia (Very Forward Medical Officer):

- Vivax
- Falciparum
- Malariae
- Ovale

P. vivax:

- Affects young RBCs (reticulocytes)
- Benign, tertian fever (fever every 3rd day; after 48 hours)
- Schuffner's dots
- Splenic rupture

P. falciparum:

- Affects all types of RBCs
- Maurer's dots
- Banana shaped gametes
- Multiple infestation of RBCs
- Malignant tertian malaria (fever every 3rd day; after 48 hours)
- Blackwater fever (Renal failure + DIC)
- Cerebral malaria

P. malariae:

- Affects mature RBCs
- Ziemann's dots
- Benign quartan fever (fever after 72 hours; every 4th day)

P. ovale:

- Rarest in India
- James dots

CHAPTER 7

FORENSIC MEDICINE

I. COURT PROCEDURES

Inquest:

- Investigation into cause of death (conducted in cases of murder, suicide, accidents & suspicious deaths): Inquest/ judicial inquiry
- CrPC 174 deals with inquest
- In case of death in lock-up, inquest is carried out by: Executive Magistrate (Collector, Deputy collector, Tahsildar etc.)

Magistrate inquest is done in:

- Death in police custody
- Death in police firing
- Death in mental asylum
- Death in prison
- Exhumation
- Dowry death

Terms related to courts of Law:

- Cognizable/ grave offences: Police officer can arrest without an arrest warrant (Murder, Rape etc.)
- Written document issued by the court (served on the witness under a penalty in all cases by the police officer to attend the court for giving evidence on a particular day & time): Subpoena/ summon
- Fee paid to a witness at the time of serving summons (to cover the expenses for attending the court): Conduct money (given only in civil case)
- Telling lies by a witness under oath OR Failure to tell what he knows/ believes to be true: Perjury (section 191 IPC)
- A leading question is one which includes the material facts and suggests to the witness, the answer desired and admits of a conclusive answer by YES or NO
- Leading questions are allowed during cross-examination.
- Mental ability to make a valid will: Testamentary capacity
- McNaughten's rule is for: Criminal responsibility of the insane;
- Dying declaration: Written/ oral statement of a person, who is dying, due to some unlawful act, relating to his death
- Dying deposition: A magistrate records the statement
- Expert witness: Person who is qualified/ experienced in a scientific/ technical subject like
    - o Doctor,
    - o Firearm expert,
    - o Finger print expert
- In India, a death sentence can be commuted (exchange a penalty for a less severe one) by: President
- Amnesty (the formal act of liberating someone) for capital punishment vest (have power & authority) with: President

Exhumation

- Exhumation is done after a written order from: 1st class judicial magistrate
- It is conducted in: Day-light (so started in early morning)
- Maximum time limit for exhumation in India: NO time limit

Magistrates:

- Punishment by a Chief judicial magistrate: Sentence of imprisonment upto 7 year
- Punishment by a judicial magistrate of 1st class (C):
  - o 3 years imprisonment
  - o Fine up to 10,000
- Second class judicial magistrate:
  - o Imprisonment up to 1 year
  - o Fine up to 5000 rupees

II. MEDICAL JURISPRUDENCE

Some important IPCs:

- 193: Punishment of false evidence (perjury)
- 197: Signing/ issuing false certificates
- 300: Murder
- 302: Punishment for murder
- 304A: Causing death by negligence
- 304B: Dowry death
- 319: Definition of hurt
- 320: Grievous hurt
- 321: Voluntarily causing hurt
- 354: Assault to outrage the modesty of a woman
- 375: Definition of Rape
- 376: Punishment of Rape
- 497: Adultery

Some terms:

- Professional secrecy: The doctor obliged to keep secret all things about his patient, which he comes to know during his professional work.
- Privileged communication: Statement communicated by a doctor to concerned authorities to protect the interests of community. Examples:
  - o A person with some infectious disease working as a cook
  - o A Engine/ bus driver found to be colour blind
  - o Syphilitic taking bath in a public pool
- Novus actus interveniens: A doctor is responsible for his actions & also for its consequences. It means an unrelated action intervening. Example:
  - o A doctor leaving a scissor or swab in the abdomen, he becomes negligent.
- Professional negligence/ Malpraxis: It is the absence of reasonable care & skill or willful negligence on part of a doctor, which may result in injury or death of the patient
- Therapeutic misadventure: Case in which a patient is injured or dies due to some unintentional act done by a doctor or hospital
- Contributory negligence: It is the negligence of the patient, combined with the doctor's negligence, which contributes to the injury as a direct cause and without which the injury would not have occurred.
- Vicarious liability: An employer is responsible not only for his negligence but also for the negligence of his employees, if such negligence occurs in course of employment and within its scope, by the principle of respondent superior (let the master answer)
- Res ipsa loquitor: It means things speak for itself.
- Euthanasia/ Mercy killing: It means causing painless death to a person suffering from hopelessly incurable and painful disease

III. IDENTIFICATION

Some important terms:

- Corpus delicti: Elements of any criminal offence; body of offence, essence of crime. Example murder

Determination of race:

- Cephalic index/ CI: Maximum breadth of skull X 100/ Maximum length of skull
  - o Short headed/ brachycepahlic: CI of 80-85 (Mongoloids)
  - o Mesaticephalic/ medium headed: CI of 75-80 (Indians)
  - o Dolicocephalic/ long headed: CI of 70-75 (Aryans, Negroes)

- From hair: Non-fragmented medulla in Negroids

Determination of age:

- Secondary sexual characteristics
- Teeth:
  - o It is a best/ most precise method to study age up to: 14 years
  - o Temporary/ deciduous teeth: 20 in number in each jaw
  - – 4 incisors
  - – 2 canines
  - – 4 molars
  - o Factor delaying dentition:
  - – Hypothyroidism/ Cretinism (MC),
  - – Ill-nourished,
  - – Rickets
  - – GH deficiency
  - o Eruption of primary teeth is completed by: 2 to 2.5 years
  - o Mixed dentition is seen in: 6-12 years (total number of teeths are 24)
  - o First permanent molar appears at: 6 years
- Gustafsons method: Age estimation of adult over 25 years depending upon physiological age changes in dental tissue
  - o Secondary dentine
  - o Cementum apposition
  - o Root resorption
  - o Attrition
  - o Paradentosis
  - o Translucency (most reliable of all parameters)

Dactylography/ Fingerprint system/ Dermatoglyphics:

- Study of fingerprints is known as: Galton system/ Dermatoglyphics
- Most reliable method of identification of a person
- The fingerprint is unique to an individual.
- Adolphe Quetlets rule of biological variation: Even 2 identical twins don't have identical finger prints
- MC type of fingerprints: Loops (67%)
- In India, left thumb impression is taken in males as most of the males do manual work with right hand so there may be injury scars.
- Permanent loss of finger prints occur in:
  - o Leprosy
  - o Electrical injury
  - o Radiation injury

Other methods of identification:

- Chelioscopy: Study of prints of lips
- Poroscopy: Further study of finger prints utilizing study of pores
- Podogram: Footprints
- Superimposition: A technique in identifying a person by superimposing the X-ray of the skull found after death on the photo of the face of the person

Bone age estimation

- Fusion of different landmarks:
  - o Xiphoid unites with the body of sternum at 40 years of age
  - o Anterior fontanelles close & the two halves of the mandible unite at the 2nd years
  - o Closure of all sutures of the skull indicate that the age is more than 60 years
  - o Sacrum becomes a single bone by 20 to 25 year
- Angle of Mandible: Obtuse (140 degree) in old age & children
- Rule of Haase for age estimation of fetus:
  - o Up to 5 months: Age of fetus is square root of length of fetus in cm
  - o After 5 months: Length in cm/ 5 gives age in months

IV. POST-MORTEM CHANGES

Signs of immediate somatic death:

- Insensibility & loss of voluntary power (earliest sign)
- Cessation of circulation
- Cessation of respiration

Algor mortis:

- Cooling of body after death
- Most useful single indicator for postmortem interval during the first 24 hours after death
- Rate of fall of temperature is 0.5 degree Celsius per hour
- Internal organs take 24 hours to cool

Post mortem caloricity:

- Temperature remains high for the first 2 hours
- Example:
  - o Disturbance of heat regulation: Sun-stroke
  - o Increased production of heat due to muscular activity: Tetanus
  - o Excessive bacterial activity: Septicemia

Post-mortem hypostasis/ lividity/ staining/ livor mortis:

- Early sign of death
- It starts as: Blotchy discoloration
- Bluish purple or purplish red discoloration, which appears under the skin of the dependent part of the body after death due to capillovenous distension.
- Usually well developed within 4 hours & reaches a maximum between 6 and 12 hours
- Conditions & color:
  - o Carbon monoxide poisoning: Cherry red
  - o Hydrocyanic acid poisoning: Bright red

Rigor mortis:

- Stiffening of muscles with shortening of the fibers
- It develops within 3 hours after death
- In India: begins 1 to 2 hour hours after death & takes further 1 to 2 hours to develop
- Muscles affected in rigor mortis: All muscles (voluntary/ involuntary)
- Order of appearance: Involuntary muscles of myocardium > upper eyelids > ...... > lower limb muscle (Disappears in same order)
- Follows rule of 12:
  - o 12 hours to set in
  - o 12 hours to pass off

Cadaveric spasm:

- In this condition, the muscles that are contracted during life, become stiff and rigid immediately after death, without the stage of primary relaxation
- Usually limited to a single group of muscles and usually involves hand
- Seen mainly in voluntary muscles
- Seen in:
  - o Asphyxia deaths
  - o Brain injury
  - o Cerebral hemorrhage
  - o Drowning

Putrefaction:

- Final stage following death, produced mainly by the action of bacterial enzymes, mostly anaerobic organism derived from the bowel.
- Clostridium welchii produces lecithinase
- First sign of putrefaction externally: Greenish discoloration (because of sulphmethemoglobin) of skin over caecum (right iliac fossa)
- First sign of putrefaction internally: Reddish brown discoloration of the inner surface of the vessels, especially the aorta
- Marbling is prominent in 36 to 48 hours
- Last organ to putrefy in males:
  - o Prostate,
  - o Testis
- Last organ to putrefy in females:
  - o Non-gravid uterus,
  - o Ovaries
- Bone is the last structure is putrefy in both males & females
- Caspers dictum: A body decomposes in air twice as rapidly as in water and eight times as rapid as in earth.
- Putrefaction is rapid in damp, marshy and shallow graves
- Putrefactive changes in liver:
  - o Honey combing,
  - o Foamy liver

- Putrefaction is delayed by (poisons):
  - o Arsenic
  - o Carbolic acid
  - o ZnCl
  - o Strychnine

Saponification/ Corpse wax:

- It is seen in body immersed in water or damp warm environment
- Adipocere formation is also known as: Saponification
- Climate for adipocere formation:
  - o Warm
  - o Moisture
  - o Humid
- Biochemically Adipocere formation is: Hydrolysis & hydrogenation of pre-existing fat

Mummification:

- Modification of putrefaction
- Body is odourless
- Seen when the body is buried in dry sandy shallow graves
- Mummification is:
  - o Dessication,
  - o Dehydration,
  - o Shrinkage of cadaver (preserving body features)
- Mummification is seen in:
  - o Dry air condition
  - o Free air circulation around the body
  - o Wind
  - o High temperature, lack of moisture

V. INJURIES

Abrasions:

- Destruction of the skin, involving superficial layers of epidermis only
- MC type of abrasions: Graze
- Brush burn:
  - o A type of graze
  - o Caused by violent lateral rubbing by friction force
  - o Fall while running (dragging over ground)
- Patterned/ pressure/ imprint abrasion: Pressure injury caused by crushing of the superficial layers of the epidermis

Bruises:

- An effusion of blood into the tissues, due to the rupture of the subcutaneous vessels, caused by violence
- Blue colour of bruise is due to: Deoxyhemoglobin
- Green colour of bruise is due to: Haematoidin
- Artificial bruises: some irritant substances when rubbed on skin produces injuries resembling bruises. Example:
  - o Semicarpus anacardium (marking nut)
  - o Calotropis
- Age of bruise:
  - o Blue colour of bruise is seen after: Few hours to 3 days
  - o 4th day: Bluish black to brown (hemosiderin)
  - o Green colour of bruise is seen at: 5 to 6 days
  - o 7 to 12th day: Yellow (bilirubin)
  - o 2 weeks: Normal

Incised wounds/ IW:

- IW is clean cut throughout tissues, which is longer than deep
- Towards the end of the cut, the wound becomes shallow (tailing of the wound) and it indicates direction of the injury.
- Tentative cuts/ Hesitation marks: Suicidal attempts
- Healing of clean, incised wound is by: Primary intention
- Gaping of wound is determined by: Langer's lines

Lacerated wounds/ LW:

- They are tears of skin, mucus membranes, muscle or internal organs produced by application of blunt force to the broad area of the body.

- There is characteristic tissue bridges present in LW
- Margins are irregular with abrasions in LW as compared to IW
- Incised looking wounds/ incised lacerated wound: Lacerated wounds look like incised wounds, especially seen on
  - o Scalp
  - o Eyebrows
  - o Cheekbones
  - o Lower jaw
  - o Iliac crest

Stab/ puncture wound:

- Depth is maximum in: Stab wound
- Fish tailing is seen if a single edged weapon is used. One angle of the wound will be sharp, the other would be torn or blunt

Regional injuries:

- Fracture a la signature/ Depressed fracture:
  - o Outer table of skull driven into diploe,
  - o Inner table is fractured irregularly
  - o Due to heavy object with small striking area like axe, hammer etc.
- Pond fracture/ ping-pong ball fracture/ Indented fracture:
  - o Indented fracture of elastic skull
  - o Seen in skulls of infant
- Gutter fracture: Oblique bullet wound, removing a part of the thickness of the bone forming a gutter
- Contrecoup lesions: Injury is present in an area opposite to the side of impact in head injury.

Motor vehicle related injuries:

- Whiplash injury: Hyperflexion followed by hyperextension of cervical spine
- Seatbelt injury: MC causes rupture of small bowel and associated injury to mesentery
- Bumper fracture: Wedge shaped fracture of tibia & fibula if the vehicle hits from behind
- Sparrow's foot marks: Bizarre shaped lacerations that develops when the face comes in contact with shattered windshield glass

Firearm injuries:

- Choking (firearm): Constricting device at the muzzle end of a shotgun. Purpose is to lessen the rate of shot after it leaves the muzzle
- Bevelling of the skull in bullet injury:
  - o In entry wound: On inner table of skull
  - o In exit wound: On the outer table
- Contents of black gun powder:
  - o 75% Potassium nitrate (oxidizing agent)
  - o 10% Sulfur (binding agent)
  - o 15% Charcoal (fuel)
- Smokeless powder:
  - o Single base: Nitrocellulose
  - o Double base: Nitroglycerine & nitro-cellulose
  - o Triple base: Nitroglycerine & nitro-cellulose with Nitro guanidine
- Tandem bullets: 2 bullets in succession
- Dumdum bullet: Tip is chiseled out, which fragments extensively upon striking.
- Abraded collar/ Grease collar/ Dirt collar:
  - o Entrance wound of gun shot/ bullet injury
  - o Tells us about the direction
- Paraffin wax test/ Dermal nitrate test/ Diphenyl Amine test detects: Gun powder/ gun shot residues on hands of the person who has fired the gun

Grievous hurt:

- Emasculation (sterility/ impotency)
- Permanent privation/ loss of sight of one or both eyes
- Permanent privation/ loss of hearing from one or both ears
- Privation/ loss of any member or joint
- Destruction/ Permanent impairing of power of any member or joint
- Permanent disfigurement of the head or face
- Fracture/ dislocation of a bone or tooth
- Any hurt which endangers life or which causes the victim to be in severe bodily pain or unable to follow his ordinary pursuits for a period of 20 days.

VI. ASPHYXIAL DEATHS

Burking:

- It is a method of
  - o Homicidal smothering (closing the external respiratory opening by hand) &
  - o Traumatic asphyxia (sitting on chest)
  - o Named after William Burk

Hanging:

- Constricting force in hanging: Weight of the body
- Partial hanging:
  - o Bodies are partially suspended
  - o Weight of the head acts as the constricting force
- Typical hanging: Ligature forms the from the midline above the thyroid cartilage symmetrically on either side of the neck to the occipital region
- Atypical hanging: When the knot is placed at site other than that seen in typical hanging
- Le facies sympathique:
  - o Knot presses the cervical sympathetic trunk, the eye on that side remain open & the pupil is dilated
  - o Indicates antemortem hanging
- Ligature marks are a type of: Printed abrasion
- Saliva may be found dribbling from the angle of mouth (sure sign) on the opposite side of the knot.
- MC site of fracture hyoid: Junction of inner two-third and outer one-third of greater cornua

Judicial hanging:

- Cause of death in judicial hanging: Fracture dislocation at C2-C3 (dens) or rarely C3-C4
- Knot is placed below chin
- Cause of death: Brainstem damage

Café coronary/ Food asphyxia:

- Accidental choking
- Victim may be observed collapsing on the dining table suddenly without any signs of respiratory distress
- It appears as if the victim died because of MI. Hence called cafe coronary
- Autopsy will reveal a bolus of food in the pharynx or larynx
- Café coronary is common in:
  - o Mostly overdrunk
  - o Deeply intoxicated
  - o With depressed gag reflex
- Cause of death in café coronary: Asphyxia/ Reflex cardiac arrest from stimulation of vagus (laryngeal nerve)

Drowning:

- Signs of drowning:
  - o Fine copious, persistent, white, frothy discharge from mouth & nose,
  - o Diatoms in bone marrow & brain (suggest antemortem drowning),
  - o Goose skin/ cutis anserine in which the has granular and puckered appearance
  - o Washer woman's hand: Wrinkling of limbs indicate that body was in water.
- MC type of drowning: Accidental
- Gettlers test is done for: Drowning (differentiate fresh water & sea water drowning)
- Substance estimated in Gettlers test:
  - o Chloride content of the blood in both sides of heart
  - o In fresh water drowning, chloride content of the left side of the heart is 50% lower
  - o In sea water drowning, chloride content of the left side of the heart is higher.
- Typical drowning:
  - o Wet/ primary drowning
  - o Water is inhaled into lungs
  - o Cause of death:
    - – Sea water: Cardiac arrest/ asystole
    - – Fresh water: Ventricular fibrillation
- Emphysema aquosum: In wet drowning the lungs are over distended and alveolar walls are torn

- Edema aquosum: Seen in drowning of unconscious/ postmortem drowning
- Diatoms/ Bacillariophyceae:
  - o Unicellular silica coated algae, suspended in water
  - o Their presence in bone marrow & brain signifies drowning
  - o Most common used bone is sternum

VII. THERMAL INJURIES

Lightning stroke:

- Arborescent burns:
  - o Filigree burns/ Litchenberg's flowers/ Keraunographic markings
  - o Superficial, irregular, thin & resembles branches of a tree
- Flash of lightning is due to an electrical discharge from a cloud to the earth

Electrical burns:

- Joule burns: Electricity burns (entry point of the current)
- Crocodile skin appearance of skin: Suggestive of high voltage electric burns (causes large areas of skin damage)

BURNS

Degree of burns:

- Epidermal:
  - o First & second degree
  - o Usually a blister
  - o Very painful
  - o Repair is complete without scar formation
- Dermo-epidermal:
  - o Third & fourth degree
  - o Whole thickness of skin is destroyed
  - o Most painful
- Deep:
  - o Fifth & sixth degree
  - o Gross destruction not only of the skin & subcutaneous tissue but also of muscle & even bone
  - o Nerve endings are also destroyed and as such, the burns are relatively painless

Features of antemortem burns:

- Line of redness present (absent in postmortem burns)
- Blister contain serous fluid with chloride & albumin (Postmortem vesicles contains air)
- Soot in upper respiratory passage (absent in postmortem burns)
- More than 5% carboxyhemoglobin in blood (less in postmortem burns)
- Increase in enzyme reaction
- Presence of vital reactions (not increased in post mortem burns)

Pugilistic attitude:

- Pugilistic/ boxing/ defensive attitude is due to which process: Protein coagulation (causes stiffening in this attitude)
- Coagulation of protein albumin of the muscles which cause contraction and thus pugilistic attitude
- Pugilistic attitude is seen after: Burns (both antemortem & postmortem)

Heat hematoma:

- Resembles extradural hemorrhage
- Most common site is parieto-temporal region
- Occurs between skull & duramater

VIII. TOXICOLOGY

Universal antidote (ATM):

- Animal charcoal:
  - o 2 parts
  - o Absorbs alkaloids
- Tannic acid:
  - o 1 part
  - o Precipitates alkaloids
- Magnesium oxide:
  - o 1 part
  - o Neutralizes acid without gas formation

METALLIC POISONS

Chronic mercury poisoning:

-
- Features:
  - o Erethism:
    - – Seen in persons working with mercury in mirror manufacturing firms
    - – Neuro-psychiatric manifestations: Irritability, shyness, mental depression, loss of memory & insomnia
  - o Shaking palsy/ Hatter's shake/ glass blowers shake:
    - – Coarse, intentional tremors
  - o Mercurial lentis:
    - – Brown deposit of mercury through cornea on the anterior lens capsule
  - o Acrodynia/ Pink disease:
    - – Acro means limbs; odynia means pain
    - – Hands & feet becomes puffy, pinkish, painful & paresthetic
  - o Hydrar gyrism:
    - – Fine tremors of the tongue, hands, arms etc.
- Acute mercury poisoning mainly involves: Kidney (PCT) causes proximal renal tubular necrosis
- Minimata disease: Contamination of fish with mercury (in Minimate Bay, Japan)

Arsenic poisoning:

- Findings on nails:
  - o Aldrich Mee's lines/ leuko-paronychia
  - o Transverse lines on nails
- 2 types of presentation:
  - o Fulminant type
  - o Gastroenteric type
- Gastroenetric type of Arsenic poisoning:
  - o MC type
  - o Mimic Cholera poisoning
  - o Stools are expelled frequently and involuntarily
  - o Initially stools are dark coloured and stinking but later on becomes colorless, odourless and watery resembling rice water stools of cholera
- Skin changes associated with arsenic poisoning:
  - o Rain drop pigmentation: Finely mottled brown changes mostly on temples, eyelids & neck
  - o Rash resembling fading Measles rash
- Appearance of hair: Golden hair
- Arsenophagists:
  - o People who can tolerate high doses of arsenic as tonic or an aphrodisiac
  - o Tolerance of up to 0.3 gm or more in one dose
- Special feature of arsenic poisoning: Retardation of putrefaction & Delayed rigor
- Arsenic can be detected in: Completely decomposed bones, charred bodies, ash, hairs & nails
- Tests for arsenic poisoning:
  - o Marsh's test
  - o Reinsch's test
  - o Gutzeit test
- Treatment:
  - o Freshly prepared precipitated hydrated ferric chloride
  - o BAL is the antidote

Lead poisoning/ plumbism/ Saturnism:

- Inhalation of lead dust & fumes by makers of white lead, smelters, plumbers, glass polishers
- Features of lead poisoning/ plumbism/ saturnism (ABCDEF):
  - o Anemia (due to decreased RBC survival)
  - o Basophilia (punctate) of RBCs (dark blue spots in cytoplasm of RBCs)
  - o Burtonian/ lead line in upper jaw
  - o Constipation & colic, Coproporphyrin in urine increased,
  - o Death, wrist Drop & foot Drop
  - o Encephalopathy (in children)
  - o Facial pallor (most consistent sign)
- Burtonian line is seen at:
  - o Appears at the gingiva-tooth border
  - o Due to lead sulphide (after prolonged high level exposure)
- Early manifestation of chronic lead poisoning: Facial pallor

- Treatment: Combination of BAL + Calcium disodium versenare

CORROSIVE POISONS

Sulphuric acid:

- Strongest corrosive poison
- Brown to black streaks from angle of mouth present
- Effect of sulphuric acid poisoning on gastric mucosa:
  - o Stomach mucosa is stained black/ scalded (Perforation of stomach is common)
  - o Blotting paper appearance of mucosa of stomach
- Fatal period for H_2SO_4: 18 to 24 hours
- Gastric lavage is contraindicated
- Vitriolage:
  - o Throwing of H_2SO_4 on other individual
  - o Comes under Sec. 320 IPC
  - o Affected part is washed with plenty of water and soap or sodium or potassium carbonate. Later a thick paste of magnesium oxide or carbonate is applied

Carbolic acid:

- Carbolic acid is also known as phenol
- Carboluria:
  - o Urine turns green or black on exposure to air/ smoky green urine
  - o In the body phenol is partially oxidized to hydroquinone and pyrocatechol.
  - o These are excreted in urine along with unchanged phenol.
  - o The further oxidation of hydroquinone and pyrocatechol in the urine causes green coloration
- Appearance of stomach in carbolic acid poisoning: Mucous membrane is thickened & looks brownish and leathery (white leathery appearance)
- Special feature of carbolic acid poisoning: Retards putrefaction

ORGANIC IRRITANT POISON

Abrus precatorius/ Ratti:

- Seeds contain an active principle, a toxalbumin 'Abrin' (abrin resembles viper snake venom)
- Used as a cattle poison by making needles (sui)

Calotropis:

- Juice is introduced into uterus on an abortion sticks (criminal abortion)
- Also used as arrow poison
- Used to produce artificial bruises

SNAKE

Snakes & nature of venom:

- Russells viper venom is: Hemolytic/ Hemotoxic/ vasculotoxic due to phosphotidase
- Cobra, Krait venom (elapidae family) is: Neurotoxic
- Sea/marine snake venom is: Myotoxic/ Marked muscle weakness/ polymyositis

CHAPTER 8

PSM

I. BIOSTATISTICS

Mean:

- Calculated as sum of all values divided by the total number of values
- For example mean of 2, 3 and 4 would be calculated as
- Take sum of 2, 3 & 4. This is 9
- Divide it by total number of values. These are 3
- 9 ÷ 3 equals to 3

Mode:

- It is the most frequently occurring value
- For example, mode of 2, 3, 4, 3 would be 3 as 3 is coming twice in the given set of numbers

Median:

- In ascending/ descending order, the middlemost value is the median if total numbers of value are odd (average of middle two values in case of even numbers)
- For example median of 2, 4, 3 would be 3 (by arranging the values in ascending order as 2, 3, 4 or in descending order as 4, 3, 2)

Standard deviation/ SD:

- 95% of values fall under: 2SD
- SD is most appropriate measure of dispersion
- SD is calculated as the RMS (root mean square) deviation of the values from the mean

Chi-square test:

- Used to compare non-continuous data in 2 groups
- Used to test significance of association between 2 or more qualitative characteristics

Simple random sampling:

- Sample is drawn in such a way that each unit has an equal chance of being drawn in a sample
- Method include lottery method, computer software etc.

Stratified random sampling:

- Population is divided to groups/ classes and sample is drawn from each group at random.

Cluster random sampling:

- Basically used for assessing immunization status of children under immunization
- 30 clusters, each containing 7 children (30 × 7 technique; total of 210 children)

Sample registration system:

- SRS is essentially a dual record system for providing quick and reliable estimates of birth and death rates on a continuous basis at national and state level separately for rural and urban areas.
- An independent half-yearly survey of births and deaths by an investigator is done

Degree of freedom:

- Calculated as (n-1) × (m-1)

- Where n is number of columns and m is number of rows
- For example degree of freedom in a contingency table of 3 × 5 would be (3-1) × (5-1) = 8

Bar diagrams/ Charts

- It is a simple diagram or a chart, popularly used to compare the magnitude of the qualitative data.
- Bars are the rectangles drawn along the graph sheet.

II. NUTRITION

Proteins:

- Protein Efficiency Ratio: Weight gain (in grams) per gram of protein intake
- Digestibility coefficient/ DC: Ratio of Nitrogen absorbed to Nitrogen consumed
- Biological value/ BV: Ratio of Nitrogen retained to Nitrogen absorbed
- Net Protein Utilization: Product of BV and DC

Xerophthalmia:

- MC in aged 1-3 years
- First clinical symptom of vitamin A deficiency: Night blindness/ nyctalopia
- Under National immunization schedule, 1 lac IU is given at 9 months of age (along with measles vaccine)

VITAMINS

Vitamin A:

- Earliest symptom of vitamin A deficiency: Night blindness/ Nyctalopia
- Earliest sign of vitamin A deficiency: Conjunctival xerosis (characteristic appearance of 'emerging like sand banks at receding tide')
- Effect of fat on absorption of vitamin A: Increases
- Vitamin A deficiency is a child health problem if prevalence of night blindness in children's aged 6 months to 6 years is: 1%
- For Bitot's spots the prevalence should be more than >0.5%

Other vitamins:

- Vitamin which prevents lipid peroxidation: Vitamin E (also vitamin A and vitamin C)
- Vitamin which is required for gamma carboxylation: Vitamin K

Iron-Folic acid supplementation:

- During pregnancy, IFA tablets contain (specific protection): 100 mg elemental iron & 500 microgram of FA (daily)
- Amount for paediatric population (under RCH): Amount is $1/5^{th}$ (20 mg elemental iron & 100 microgram of FA daily)

Egg:

- Poor in: Carbohydrate, Vitamin C
- Energy yielded from egg: 70 Kcal
- Net Protein Utilization/ NPU of hen's egg: 96

Milk:

- Skimmed milk: Fat has been removed from the milk
- Milk is a poor source of: Iron & vitamin C
- Pasteurization of milk: Rapidly heating milk, then keeping it uniformly and then allowing it to cool rapidly
- Pasteurization kills: 90% of bacteria in milk, including heat resistant tubercle bacillus & Q fever
- Pasteurization doesn't kill: Thermoduric bacteria, nor the bacterial spores
- Methods of pasteurization of milk:
  - o Holder/ Vat method (used for small and rural communities)
  - o HTST method (Most widely done procedure)
  - o HHST method
  - o UHT method
- Tests for pasteurization of milk to check adequacy:
  - o Phosphatase test (widely test)

    - Standard plate count
    - Coliform count
- Use of pasteurization: Milk can be preserved for 8 to 12 hours at 18 degree C
- Methylene blue reduction test/ MBRT in milk is done to:
    - Detection of micro-organism in the milk/ contamination of milk
    - MBRT is carried out on milk accepted for pasteurization

Cereals:

- Jaggery has high concentration of: Iron
- Ragi, dates are rich source of: Calcium
- Pulses are deficient in: Methionine (and cysteine)
- Cereals are deficient in: Threonine (& Lysine)
- Maize is deficient in: Tryptophan (& Lysine)
- Highest biological value is: Egg

FATTY ACID/ FA

Essential FA:

- Most important EFA is linoleic acid as it serve as a basis of production of EFA
- Deficiency of EFA lead to phrenoderma/ toad skin
- Example of EFA (cannot be synthesized in human body and hence to be supplied in diet):
    - Linoleic acid (PUFA),
    - Linolenic acid (PUFA)
    - Arachidonic acid
    - Eicosapentanoic acid
    - Not all EFA are PUFA (polyunsaturated fatty acids)

Rich source of linoleic acid:

- Safflower oil (73%),
- Corn oil (57%)
- Sunflower oil (56%)
- Soyabean oil (51)

Endemic fluorosis:

- Mottling of dental enamel, with chalky white appearance (Caries) best seen on upper jaw incisors at level more than 1.5 ppm
- Skeletal fluorosis at fluorine level between 3 -6 ppm
- Intervention: Nalgonda technique (NEERI, Nagpur)
  It involves addition of lime, alum and bleaching powder followed by flocculation, sedimentation and filtration.

FOOD ADULTERATION

Epidemic dropsy:

- Epidemic dropsy is due to contamination of mustard oil with: Argemone oil (containing sanguinarine)
- Biochemical Effect of sanguinarine: Interferes with oxidation of pyruvic acid, which accumulates in blood
- This lead to sudden non-inflammatory edema of lower limbs (bilateral), diarrhoea, glaucoma, cardiac failure, dyspnea and death.

Aflatoxicosis:

- Toxin: Aflatoxin
- Food stuff affected by: Aspergillus flavus

Ergotism:

- Toxin: Clavine alkaloids
- Foodstuff affected by: Claviceps fusiformis

Lathyrism:

- Toxin: Beta-Oxayl Amino Alanine/ BOAA
- Food stuff (Kesari dal) affected by: Lathyrus sativus

III. ENVIRONMENT

Sound:

- Hearing ability is measured by: Audiometer
- Tympanic membrane ruptures if the intensity of sound is more than: 150 -160 dB
- Maximum tolerable limit of sound per day is: 85 – 90 dB

Air:

- Chemical indicators of air pollution:
    - o Coefficient of haze
    - o Smoke & soiling index
    - o Best indicator is Sulphur dioxide

WATER

- Recommended fluorine concentration in water: 0.5 – 0.8 ppm (<1.5 ppm)
- Fluoride concentration: 1.5 mg/ L

Drinking water quality standards:

- E. coli or thermotolerant coliforms: Nil
- Nitrites (recent contamination): <3 mg/ L
- Nitrates (remote contamination): <50 mg/ L

Hardness of water:

Classification	Mg/ L or ppm	Grains/ Gallon
Soft	< 17.1	<1.0
Slightly hard	17.1 – 60	1.0 – 3.5
Moderately hard	60 – 120	3.5 – 7.0
Hard	120 -180	7.0 – 10.5
Very hard	>180	>10.5

Hardness of water:

- Hardness level of (mEq/ L) of hard water: 3-6 (150-300 mg/L)
- Softening of hard water:
    - o Softening is recommended at level of hardness >3 mEq/ L
    - o Permutit process is for removing temporary hardness

Water disinfection:

- Ortho-tolidine arsenite/ OTA test: Determines both free & combined chlorine
- Orthotoludine test determines: Free chlorine and total chlorine
- Total chlorine: Sum of free and combined chlorine
- Horrock's apparatus: Measures chlorine demand of water (to find out the dose of bleaching powder required for disinfection of water)

Instruments:

- Wind vane: Assess direction of air/ wind
- Kata thermometer: Assess cooling power of air & air velocity
- Sling psychrometer/ Hygrometer: Humidity
- Venturimeter: Measuring bed strength in slow sand filter
- Anemometer: Assess air/ wind velocity

IV. HEALTH CARE IN INDIA

Health care in India:

- Tertiary level of care: Medical Colleges & Hospitals
- Secondary level of care: Community health centre
- Primary level of care: Primary health centre
- Subcenter

ASHA:

- Works under NRHM mission
- Educated till VIII class

MPW:

- Multipurpose worker is present at Subcentre
- Caters to a population of 5000

VHG:

- 1 village health guide caters to a population of: 1000 rural population (Trained Birth Attendant/ TBA, Anganwadi worker/ AWW also caters to a population of 1000)
- Preferably female
- Educated upto at least VI class (same qualification for TBA, AWW, MPW)
- Trained at PHC (200 hours in 3 months)

PHC:

- Population covered by PHC in hilly/ tribal area is: 20, 000 (30,000 in plains)
- PHC has 4-6 beds
- Referral centre for 6 subcentres
- 1-2 medical officers (total staff of 15)
- Under NTCP, PHC is said to be PHC-R if:

Microscopy + Radiology facility exist

Subcenter:

- 1 subcentre caters to a population of: 5,000 in plain areas (3000 in hilly/ tribal area)
- Number of staff: 3
- Most peripheral and first contact point between community and health care system

TBA:

- A trained birth dai/ trained birth attendant caters to a population of: 1000 (rural population)
- Training at PHC, subcentre or MCH centre for 30 days (has to conduct 2 supervised deliveries)
- Duty include conducting home deliveries in aseptic manner

Community Health Centers:

- As per RCH, first referral unit is: CHC
- Number of beds in CHC: 30
- Referral centre for 4 PHCs
- Total staff of 30-13 including 4 specialists (physician, surgeon, pediatrician and gynecologist)

V. INTERNATIONAL HEALTH

Important days:

- 1st December: World AIDS day
- 1st July: Doctors day
- 31st May: No Tobacco day

Important diseases:

- Diseases under IHR (International Health Regulations):
  - o Cholera
  - o Plague
  - o Yellow fever
- Diseases under International Surveillance of WHO:
  - o Malaria
  - o Louse borne typhus fever
  - o Relapsing fever
  - o Poliomyelitis
  - o Human influenza
  - o Salmonellosis
  - o Rabies

UNICEF (United Nations Children Fund):

- Headquarter: New York, USA
- Established in: 1946
- Promoting GOBI - FFF campaign"
  - o **G**rowth chart
  - o **O**RS
  - o **B**reast feeding
  - o **I**mmunization
  - o **F**emale education
  - o **F**amily spacing
  - o **F**ood supplementation

UNESCO:

- Headquarter: Paris

FAO (Food and Agricultural Organization):

- Headquarter: Rome, Italy

WHO:

- Headquarter: Geneva, Switzerland
- Founded on: 7th April, 1948 (celebrated as World Health Day)

VI. HEALTH PROGRAMMES

ICDS Scheme (Integrated Child Development Services):

- Launched in the year: 1975
- Beneficiaries in ICDS:
  - o Women in reproductive age group
  - o Pregnant and lactating women
  - o Children below 6 years of age
- Focal point of delivery of ICDS: Anganwadi

IMNCI/ Integrated Management of Neonatal & Childhood Illness:

- Beneficiaries:
  - o Infants (2 months) to 5 years children
  - o Newborn & young infants (under 2 months of age)

NVBDCP (National Vector Borne Disease Control Programme):

- Launched in the year: 2003 -2004
- VBD includes:
  - o Malaria
  - o Dengue/ Dengue Hemorrhagic fever
  - o Chikungunya
  - o Filaria
  - o Kala-azar
  - o Japanese encephalitis

NIDDCP/ National Iodine Deficiency Disorders Control Programme:

- NGCP/ National Goitre Control Programme was launched in the year: 1962
- NGCP was renamed as NIDDCP in the year: 1992
- Level of iodization in salt at production level: 30 parts per million
- Level of iodization in salt at production level: 15 ppm

NLCP (National Leprosy Control Programme):

- Launched in: 1955
- Aims to control leprosy through:
  - o Monotherapy with Dapsone
  - o Early detection of cases

NLEP (National Leprosy Elimination Programme):

- Launched in: 1983

NPCB (National Programme for Control of Blindness):

- Launched in 1976 as 100% centrally funded programme
- NPCB cut-off for blindness: <6/60
- National Institute of ophthalmology (AIIMS) is the apex institute
- Under National Programme for Control of Blindness, vision screening for children is conducted by: School teachers
- WHO definition of blindness: Visual acuity of less than 3/60 in better eye with best possible correction (BEBPC)
- MC cause of blindness in India: Cataract

NACP/ National Aids Control Programme:

- Launched in the year:
  - o Phase I in 1992
  - o Phase II in 1999
  - o Phase III in 2007

VII. CONTRACEPTION

IUCD (Intrauterine Uterine Contraceptive Device):

- IUCD components & their effects:
  - o Copper: Affects cervical mucus making sperm motility, capacitation & survival difficult
  - o Hormones: Cervical mucus viscosity increased which prevents sperm entry into cervix. Interferes with implantation
  - o Foreign body reaction reducing chances of fertilization
- CuT 200 is inserted post-natally after: 8 weeks
- If CuT 200 is implanted in myometrium, treatment is: Hysteroscopic removal
- Complications of IUCD:
  - o MC is bleeding
  - o Second MC side effect is pain (which requires removal of IUCD)
  - o Pelvic inflammatory disease
  - o Pregnancy with IUCD in situ
  - o Ectopic pregnancy (highest with progestasert)
  - o Uterine perforation
  - o Spontaneous expulsion

Cu-T 380A:

- 380 represents surface area of copper (mm^2)
- 'A' represents silver or gold (with copper)
- CuT 380A should be replaced after every: 10 years (Others have a life of 3-5 years)

Oral Contraceptive Pills/ OCP:

- OCP of choice in lactating females: Minipill/ progesterone only pill

- After discontinuing OCP, fertility returns after: 6 months
- Adverse effects of OCPs (ABCDEFGHI):
  - o **A**ltered lipid profile
  - o **B**lood clotting/ thrombosis (cerebral/ venous), breast tenderness
  - o **C**arcinoma (breast, cervix), Cholestatic jaundice
  - o **D**epression
  - o **E**levated BP (hypertension)
  - o **F**luid retention (weight gain)
  - o **G**all bladder disease
  - o **H**epatocellular adenoma
  - o **I**nfarction (myocardial)
- Beneficial effects of OCPs (EUROPE):
  - o **E**ctopic pregnancy
  - o **U**terine/ endometrial carcinoma
  - o **R**educed chances of Iron deficiency anemia
  - o **O**varian (benign) disease/ ovarian cysts and ovarian (malignant) disease (ovarian carcinoma)
  - o **P**ID
  - o **E**ndometriosis
- Absolute contraindications for OCPs (ACTH):
  - o **A**bnormal uterine bleeding (undiagnosed)
  - o **C**ancer (breast & genital)
  - o **T**hromboembolism
  - o **H**epatic diseases

NORPLANT (Levonorgestrel):

- Subdermal implant
- 6 silastic capsules containing 35 mg levonorgestrel each
- Effective for 5 years
- Mechanism of action: Prevents ovulation

STERILIZATION

Criteria for sterilization:

- Age of male between 25-50 years and
- Age of female between 20-45 years,
- Couple should have atleast 2 living children at the time of operation

Pomeroy's method of female sterilization:

- Isthmo-ampullary portion is ligated (middle portion is formed into a loop which is tied with catgut and excised)

NSV (non-scalpel vasectomy)/ key-hole vasectomy:

- Vas is taken out through a small puncture wound and no stitches are needed after the procedure
- Surgical hook (and not scalpel) is used to enter scrotum

EMERGENCY CONTRACEPTION

Emergency contraception is by:

- OCP (Combined OCPs/ Minipills),
- CuT (must be inserted within 5 days),
- Levonorgesterol

Dosage for emergency contraception:

- OCPs with 30 microgram estrogen (4 pills immediately followed by 4 more pills after 12 hours)
- OCPs with 50 microgram estrogen (2 pills followed by 2 more pills 12 hours later)
- Minipill 75 mg (has to be taken within 72 hours)
- Mifepristone RU 486/ antiprogestin (600 mg stat within 72 hours)

Pearl Index:

- Studying effectiveness of contraception
- It is number of failures per 100 woman years (HWY) of exposure
- Calculated as:

$$\frac{\text{Total accidental pregnancies} \times 1200}{\text{Total months of exposure}}$$

VIII. VACCINES

Properties of an ideal vaccine:

- It should be stable, cheap and safe
- It should require few administrations to produce immunity

- It should be effective in all age groups
- It should be able to pass maternal immunity to fetus as well
- It should produce immunity rapidly
- It should be effective against all variants of the micro-organism
- It should provide life-long immunity

Cold chain:

- System of transportation and storage of vaccines from the point of manufacturer to the place of administration
- In India, cold chain is maintained at: +2 to +8 degree C temperature

VACCINATION

Features of live vaccines:

- Long duration of immunity
- Contains major & minor antigen
- Live vaccines are prepared from live attenuated organisms
- Single dose is sufficient to attain immunity (except oral polio virus)

Examples of live vaccine:

- BCG,
- Yellow fever (17D)
- MMR
- Typhoral/ Ty21A
- Oral polio
- Epidemic typhus
- Chicken pox

Examples of killed vaccine:

- Salk polio
- Pertusis
- Rabies
- KFD
- Killed influenza
- JE
- HBV
- Typhim Vi
- Meningococcal
- Cholera

Cell fraction/ Fragment derived vaccine:

- Hepatitis B (polypeptides)
- Meningococcal vaccine (polysaccharide antigen of cell wall)
- Pneumococcal vaccine (polysaccharide capsule)

Toxoids:

- Tetanus toxoid
- Diphtheria toxoid

Freeze dried vaccine:

- Yellow fever (should be used within 30 minutes),
- Measles (should be used within 1-4 hours)
- BCG (should be used within 3 hours)

Reconstituted vaccines:

- BCG
- Measles
- Yellow fever

Other important facts:

- Ring immunization: Given around 100 yards of a case detected
- BCG (live attenuated vaccine) is given: Intradermally
- TY21 A (vaccine) is given for: Typhoid
- Influenza vaccine is administered as: Nose drops
- HPV vaccine is: Both bivalent & quadri-valent

Vaccine & strains:

- BCG: Danish 1331
- OPV: Sabin strain
- Chicken pox: Oka strain
- Measles: Edmonston Zagreb/ Schwartz/ Moraten strains
- Mumps: Jeryll Lyn/ Leningard/ L-Zagreb/ Urabe
- Rubella: RA-27/3
- Yellow fever: 17 D
- JE: Nakayama

Contraindications of vaccines:

- All live vaccines are C/I in pregnancy except Yellow fever
- Symptomatic HIV: All live vaccines are C/I except BCG and MMR (None of the vaccine is C/I in asymptomatic HIV)
- All live vaccines are C/I in immune-suppressive and corticosteroid therapy

Vaccine C/I in pregnancy:

- MMR (live vaccines)
- Yellow fever, though contraindicated can be given under special circumstances

Supportives in vaccines:

- Preservative in DPT: Thiomersal
- Adsorbant used in DPT: Aluminium phosphate/ Aluminium hydroxide
- Preservative in Measles vaccine: Neomycin & erythromycin
- Thermostabilizer in OPV: $MgCl_2$

IMPORTANT VACCINES

OPV:

- Dose & route: 2 drops are given orally
- Given at: 6, 10 and 14 weeks

BCG:

- Dose: 0.5 ml is intradermally at left shoulder
- Given at: Birth

DPT:

- Dose & route: 0.5 ml intramuscular in lateral part of thigh
- Given at: 6, 10 and 14 weeks

Measles:

- Dose & route: 0.5 ml, subcutaneous
- Given at: 9 months

Hepatitis B:

- Dose & route: 0.5 ml, intramuscular
- Given at: 0, 1 and 6 months as per IAP (Indian Academy of Pediatrics); 6, 10 and 14 weeks as per NIS (National Immunization Schedule)

Heat sensitivity of vaccines:

- Storage temperature for most of the vaccines: +2 degree C to 8 degree C
- OPV is highly heat sensitive vaccine (should be kept in freezer; -20 degree C)
- Vaccine vial monitors (VVM) are used for potency testing of OPV

Reverse cold chain:

- Maintenance of optimum cold temperature during transport of vaccine from periphery to the laboratory for potency testing as in OPV
- Also useful for transport of stool samples

IX. STERILIZATION & DISINFECTION

Physical methods of sterilization:

- Sunlight & drying
- Dry heat
  - o Flaming
  - o Incineration
  - o Hot air oven
- Moist heat
  - o Less than 100 degree C
  - o More than 100 degree C
- Radiation
  - o Non-ionizing: Infrared rays, Ultraviolet rays
  - o Ionizing: Gamma rays, X-rays
- Filtration
  - o Candle filter
  - o Asbestos/ Seitz filter
  - o Millipore filter

Chemical methods of sterilization:

- Phenol
- Alcohol
- Aldehyde
  - o Formaldehyde
  - o Glutaraldehyde
- Halogens

- o Chlorine
- o Iodine

- Ethylene oxide: For sterilization of sutures, heart-lung machines etc.
- Quarternary ammonium compounds

Sterilization:

- Sterilization is a process by an article is made free of all living organisms including spores.

Disinfection:

- Disinfection is a process by which a non-living object is made free of all pathogenic organisms, but non-pathogenic organisms and spores are left behind.

Bacteriostatic agent:

- Agent, added to colony, inhibits growth & vice versa

Cidex:

- Endoscopes, rubber/ plastic tubes, face masks & corrugated tubes are sterilized by: Glutaraldehyde
- Cidex is: 2% glutaraldehyde

Other important points about sterilization:

- Disposable syringes are sterilized by: Gamma rays, Ethylene oxide
- Cold sterilization is by (Sterilize without increasing temperature): Gamma rays, X-rays & cosmic rays
- Vaccines are sterilized by: Heat inactivation
- Hospital dressings are best disposed of by: Incinerator (not done for sharp)
- Reidel walker coefficient: Determines germicidal efficiency of disinfectants (as compared to phenol)

Autoclaving:

- Bacterial spores are destroyed by: Autoclaving
- Attain temperature of 122 degree C under 15 lb/ sq inch pressure for 15 minutes
- Most effective for killing spores
- Used for linen, bedsheets, dressings, gloves, OT appliances, most of culture media
- Not suitable for plastic & sharp instrument
- Bacillus stearothermophilus is sterilization control

Hot air oven:

- Utilizes 180 degree C for 1 hour
- Used for lab glasswares/ glass syringes, test tubes, surgical instruments (sharp)
- Liquid paraffin, dusting powder
- It may destroy plastic/ rubber objects (mattresses)
- Biological control for adequacy of sterilization: Spores of bacillus subtilis

Formaldehyde:

- Liquid form is used for preserving anatomical specimens
- Gaseous form is employed for fumigation of operation theatres

Glutaraldehye:

- Sterilization of endoscopes, bronchoscopes and cystoscope
- Sterilization of face mask and endotracheal tube

X. COMMUNICABLE DISEASES

Biological transmission:

- Propagative: Plague bacilli in rat flea
- Cyclo-propagative: Malaria parasite in mosquito
- Cyclodevelopmental: Microfilaria in mosquito

Cleans of safe delivery:

- Employed for: Elimination of neonatal tetanus
- CLEANS include:
  - o Clean delivery surface,
  - o Clean hands (birth attendants)
  - o Clean cord cut (blade/ instrument),
  - o Clean cord tie
  - o Clean cord stump (no applicant)

Small pox/ variola

- India declared free of small pox in: April1977
- WHO declared eradication of small pox on: 08/05/1980

Typhoid/ enteric fever:

- Causative agent: Salmonella typhii
- Mode of transmission: Feco-oral
- Laboratory tests (BASU)
  - o 1st week: Blood culture
  - o 2nd week: Antibodies
  - o 3rd week: Stool culture
  - o 4th week: Urine test
- Features: Pea-soup diarrhea
- Treatment:
  - o Cases: Quinolones (Ciprofloxacin)
  - o Carriers: Ampicillin

Chicken pox:

- Incubation period/ IP: 14-16 days
- Infectivity of chicken pox lasts for:
  - o 1 day before rash
  - o 6 days after onset of rash
- Features: Rash is pleomorphic (all stages of the rash i.e. papules, pustules, vesicles may be present at one time)
- Reactivation occurs in 10-30% results in Shingles/ Herpes zoster (Shingles is the MC late complication)
- Secondary attack rate: 90%
- Don't give Aspirin: Risk of Reye's syndrome

Diphtheria:

- Incubation Period: 2-6 days
- Caused by: Corynebacterium diphtheria
- Mode of infection: Droplet infection
- For susceptibility: Schick test

Measles/ rubeola:

- Caused by: RNA paramyxo virus (measles virus)
- Special feature in oral cavity: Kopliks spot
- Incubation period: 10 days (range 10-14 days)
- Rash appears on:
  - o 4th day after onset of fever
  - o 14th day from exposure
- Period of communicability: 4th day before rash to 5 days before rash
- Rare complication of measles: SSPE
- Protective effect of measles vaccine is exerted within: 11-12 days after administration & persist throughout life
- Contamination of measles vaccine can cause/ same vial is used after 4 hours: TSS (toxic shock syndrome)
- Features: It shows cyclical trend (cases occur every 2-3 years)
- Measles virus cannot survive outside human body
- Secondary attack rate: >80%
- No carriers
- For eradication: 95% of population must be vaccinated
- MC complication: Otitis media

Cholera:

- IP: 1-2 days
- Caused by: Vibrio cholera
- Feature: Rice water stool
- Essential part of treatment: Oral Rehydration Solution
- Chemoprophylaxis: Tetracycline
- Drug of choice in adults: Doxycyline
- Drug of choice in children: Cotrimoxazole
- Drug of choice in pregnancy: Furazolidone

Rubella:

- Incubation period: 14-21 days
- Risk to fetus is maximum if mother gets infected during: 6-12 weeks of pregnancy
- Congenital rubella syndrome:
  - o Deafness (most common if mother affected in second trimester),
  - o Cardiac malformations/ PDA (most common if mother is affected in first trimester)
  - o Cataracts
- Recommended vaccination strategy to prevent congenital rubella syndrome:

- o 1. 15-34/39 year women
  - o 2. Interrupt transmission of rubella by vaccinating all children 1-14 years
  - o 3. All children under 1 years of age
- Caused by ssRNA virus (Rubivirus)
- Mild rashes noticed on 3rd day of fever (3rd day measles) and characteristic posterior auricular, posterior cervical and occipital adenitis
- Forchheimers spots: Discrete rose coloured spots over soft palate
- Secondary attack rate: 90%

Rabies/ hydrophobia:

- Symptoms appear in: About 10 days (4 days – 8 weeks)
- IP Depends on:
  - o Site of bite
  - o Severity of the bite
  - o Number of wounds
  - o Amount of virus injected
  - o Species of biting animal
  - o Protection provided by clothing & treatment taken
- Test used for diagnosing Rabies: Antigen detection using immunoflourescence of skin biopsy
- Vaccine recommended by WHO: HDC vaccine should be replaced by cultures of animal cell lines (fetal bovine kidney, chick embryo fibroblast)
- Post exposure schedule (cell culture vaccine): HDC vaccine
  - o For unimmunized: 6 doses
  - – 0, 3, 7, 14, 28 days
  - – Booster on 90th day
  - o For immunized:
  - – 0, 3 & 7 days
- Pre-exposure:
  - o HDCV 1 ml given as I/M injection
  - o 0,7 & 28 days
- Caused by: Lyssavirus type I
- In 80% of cases, pain & tingling at the site of bite is the only symptom
- Exaggerated reflexes with hydrophobia (pathognomonic)
- Rabies is not seen in Andaman-Nicobar and Lakshadweep
- Neutralizing antibodies are present in serum/ CSF after 8th day (considered as an index of protection against infection with rabies virus)
- Dead end infection
- Street virus:
  - o Naturally occurring cases of Rabies
  - o Incubation period: 20-60 days
  - o Long & variable incubation period
  - o Forms Negri bodies
  - o Multiplication in extra-neural tissues
  - o Not used for vaccine production
- Fixed virus:
  - o Incubation period: 4-6 days
  - o Negri bodies are not formed
  - o Used for vaccine production

Yellow fever/ YF:

- Caused by: Flavivirus
- Status in India: Absent (virus is absent)
- In YF, quarantine is done for: 6 days
- Incubation period: 3-6 days
- Aedes aegyptii index is kept below 1% at sea ports & in towns for eradication in yellow fever/ endemic control
- Reservoir of infection in urban areas: Man and Aedes aegyptii
- 400 meter belt is kept free of vector breeding around ports
- Efficacy of YF vaccine starts 10 days after vaccination & lasts for 10 years

Polio:

- IM injections & tonsillectomy should be avoided during polio epidemic because: Risk of paralytic polio increases
- Cause of death in polio: Respiratory paralysis
- Pulse polio was introduced in India in: 1995
- Pulse polio is given to children below: 5 years
- A country is said to be polio FREE if there is no case confirmed for last: 3 years

- In AFP/ acute flaccid paralysis, examination for residual paralysis should be done after: 60 day
- Incubation period/ IP: 3-35 days
- P1 virus: MC cause of epidemics
- P2 virus: Most antigenic & easily eradicable
- P3 virus: MC cause of vaccine associated paralytic polio
- Infectious material: Oropharyngeal secretions & faeces
- For every clinical case, there are 1000 subclinical cases in childrens and 75 subclinical cases in adults
- History of fever at onset of paralysis is suggestive of polio
- Recommended method of confirmation of paralytic polio: Isolation of wild polio from stool

Influenza:

- Caused by orthomyxovirus (A, B & C)
- MC cause of outbreaks/ epidemics and only cause of pandemic: Type A
- H1N1: Swine flu
- H5N1: Avian flue/ Bird flu
- Cyclical trend
- Incubation Period: 18-72 hours
- Vaccines for influenza:
  - o Live attenuated
  - o Killed (may be associated with Guillain Barre syndrome)
- Swine flu is caused by: H1N1 virus
- Bird/ Avian flu is caused by: H5N1
- Drug of choice / DOC for avian influenza/ Bird flu and Swine flu is Oseltamivir/ Tamiflu
- Antigenic Drift is:
  - o Minor change/ point mutation/ small mutations in H & N
  - o Gradual/ insidious in nature
  - o Leads to sporadic cases

Hookworm:

- Ancylostoma duodenale & Necator Americana
- Chandler's index: Average number of hookworm eggs/ gram of stool
- Hookworm infestation is a major health problem if the Chandler's index is more than: 300
- Hookworm infestation causes deficiency of: Iron (as there is blood loss of 0.03-0.2 ml/ worm/ day)

HIV:

- Subtype most prevalent in India: C (HIV-I)
- Seroconversion takes: 2-12 weeks
- MC mode of transmission of HIV: Heterosexual mode (male to female is more)
- Risk of transmission by accidental needle prick: 0.3%
- Retroviral sequence in host cell: RNA-DNA-RNA
- p24 antigen disappears after: 6-8 weeks of HIV infection
- Cells attacked in HIV: CD4 cells
- CD4: CD8 ratio is: Reversed
- Window period: Time period between infection to appearance of antibodies in serum
- During window period, both ELISA & western blot are: Negative
- MC opportunistic infection in a AIDS patient in world: P. carinii
- MC opportunistic infection in a AIDS patient in India: Mycobacterium TB
- MTCT (Mother To Child Transmission) can be reduced by: Zidovudine, intrapartum nevirapine & LSCS

Pertusis/ whooping cough:

- Media used: Bordet Gengou
- Incubation Period: 1-2 weeks
- Caused by Bordetella pertusis
- Secondary attack rate: More than 90%
- Mode of transmission: Droplet
- Managed by: Erythromycin

Brucellosis/ Malta fever/ Undulant fever/ Mediterranean fever:

- Most virulent and invasive species: B. melitensis
- Reservoir: Cattle, sheep, goats

- Mode of transmission: Contact
- Contact infection occurs with direct contact with infected tissues, blood urine, vaginal discharge
- IP: 1-3 weeks
- Test done:
  - o Rose Bengal Card test,
  - o Milk ring test
- Drug of Choice/ DOC: Tetracycline

DENGUE

DF/ Dengue fever/ Break bone fever:

- Dengue is transmitted by (vector): Aedes aegypti (prefers stagnant water)
- IP: 5-6 days
- High grade fever with chills, muscle and joint pains, intense headache, retro-orbital pain, skin rash

Dengue hemorrhagic fever/ DHF:

- IP: 4-6 days
- Moderate to marked thrombocytopenia (<1 lakh/ cmm)
- Hemorrhagic manifestations
- Positive tourniquet test (>20 petechiae/ sq. inch)
- Hemoconcentration/ rising hematocrit
- Plus all features of DF

Dengue shock syndrome:

- Dengue hemorrhagic fever and shock
- Features of shock include low BP, tachycardia, Narrow pulse pressure, cold & clammy skin

MALARIA

Human cycle of plasmodium:

- Pre-erythrocytic schizogony: No clinical manifestations
- Erythrocytic schizogony: Clinical attack of malaria
- Gametogony
- Exo-erythrocytic schizogony: Causes relapse; seen in P. vivax & P. ovale

Mosquito cycle of plasmodium:

- Completion of gametogony
- Sporogomy: Mosquito are capable of transmitting the infection

Man in malaria:

- Intermediate/ secondary host
- Asexual phase
- Schizogony (pre-erythrocytic, erythrocytic & exo-erythrocyctic)

Malariometric measures:

- API/ annual parasitic index: Measure of malaria incidence
- ABER/ annual blood examination rate: Operational efficiency in malaria
- Spleen rate: Measure endemicity of malaria
- IPR/ infant parasite rate: Most sensitive index of recent malaria transmission

Other important points:

- Size of RBC is increased in: Vivax malaria
- Infective agent of malaria is: Sporozoite, transmitted through bite of an female anopheline mosquito
- Not seen in peripheral blood smear of falciparum: Schizont

TUBERCULOSIS

Tuberculosis:

- Mycobacterium TB was discovered by: Robert Koch
- Prevalence of TB in community is assessed by: Tuberculin test/ Mantoux test
- Standard dose of PPD for Mantoux test: 1 TU
- Ghon focus is related to: Primary pulmonary TB
- Ocular lesion associated with primary TB: Phylectenular conjunctivitis
- Characteristic lesion of primary TB: Fibrocaseous lesion
- Category II of DOTS includes: Previously treated smear positive (relapse, failure, default)

- Defaulter is: Has not taken drugs for more than 2 months consecutively any time after starting treatment
- Case finding in RNTCP is based on: Sputum microscopy
- Sputum smear are stained for AFB with Zeihl Neelson stain
- Other tests:
  - PCR/ NAAT test: Extremely sensitive
  - BACTEC radiometric system: 95% sensitivity
  - MMR/ mass miniature radiography: Not used now
- DOTS means: Short term treatment under supervision; Alternate day treatment given

Tuberculin test:

- Tuberculin is purified protein derivative
- 0.1 ml of 1TU PPD is injected intra-dermally on forearm & read after 72 hours
- Estimates prevalence of TB infection
- A positive test (induration >9 mm) indicates past/ present exposure/ infection by M. tuberculosis
- Prognostic significance

LEPROSY/ HANSEN'S DISEASE

Leprosy:

- Spreads by: Droplet infection
- Contact transmission:
  - Skin to skin contact
  - Contact with soil/ fomites
- Leprosy is a public health problem when prevalence is: 1:10,000
- Elimination level of leprosy: Less than 1 cases per 10,000
- India achieved level of elimination of leprosy
- Classification system/ index related to leprosy:
  - Ridley Joplings classification (BI: Counting number of bacilli in average microscopic fields)
  - Diagnosis of leprosy under National Leprosy

Elimination Programme/ NLEP (Clinical basis):

- PBL (Pauci-Bacillary leprosy): 1-5 skin lesions
- MBL (Multi-Bacillary Leprosy): More than 5 skin lesions

Operational classification (for chemo-therapy):

- Paucibacillary: <2 skin lesion
- Multibacillary: >2 skin lesions

MBL:

- Managed by 3 drugs (RDC)
- Duration: 12 months
- Annual follow up till: 5 years

PBL:

- Managed by 2 drugs (RD)
- Duration: 6 months
- Annual follow up for: 2 years

Dosage of drugs:

- Rifampicin/ R: 600 mg once a month, supervised
- Dapsone/ D: 100 mg daily
- Clofazimine/ C: 300 mg once a month, supervised

Plague/ Black sickness/ Mahamari

- Wild rodents are reservoir of infection
- Infected rodents, fleas and pneumonic plague cases are source of infection
- Rat flea (Xenopsylla cheopsis) is the most efficient vector
- Bite of an infected flea or droplet infection (pneumonic plague) is the mode of transmission
- MC type of plague is bubonic plague (2-7 days)
- Streptomycin is drug of choice
- Tetracycline is chemoprophylactic agent of choice
- Destruction of rat flea is the most effective way of breaking transmission of plague
- Causative agent of plague: Yersinia pestis (Gram negative, non-motile, cocco-bacillus)

- Staining done in a case of plague: Wayson's staining
- Most contagious type of plague: Pneumonic plague (1-2 days)
- Complication of bubonic-septicaemic plague
- IP: 1-3 days
- Specific flea index: Average number of fleas of each species/ rodent
- Best indicator of potential explosiveness of plague outbreak: Specific flea index

Rickettsial diseases:

- Brill Zinsser disease is: Recrudescent form/ Delayed manifestation of epidemic typhus/ louse borne typhus
- Vector for Epidemic typhus (R. prowazeki): Louse
- Reservoirs are humans
- Endemic/ murine typhus (R. typhi):
  - o Vector: Rat flea
  - o Rodents are the reservoir
- Scrub typhus (R. tsutsugmashi):
  - o Vector: Trombiculide Mite
  - o Rodents are the reservoir

Agents of some other Rickettsial diseases:

- Rickettsial pox: Rickettsia akari (vector is mite)
- Rocky Mountains potted fever: R. rickettsii (vector is tick)
- Trench fever: Bartonella quintana (vector is louse)
- Q fever: Coxiella burnettii (No vector)

Echinococcus granulosus/ Dog tapeworm:

- Intermediate host: Sheep
- Intermediate dead-end host: Man
- Definitive host: Dog
- Drug of choice: Albendazole

XI. NON-COMMUNICABLE DISEASES

Cancer:

- Most common cancer in males in India: Oropharyngeal cancer
- Most common cancer in males causing death in India & Worldwide: Lung cancer
- Most common cancer in males Worldwide: Lung cancer
- Most common cancer in females in India: Cervical cancer
- Most common cancer in females Worldwide: Breast cancer
- Most common cancer in females causing death in India & Worldwide: Breast cancer

Obesity:

- Indices for obesity:
  - o BMI (Quetlet's index)
  - o BMI = Weight (in Kg)/ Height^2 (in metre)
  - o Underweight: <18.5
  - o Normal: 18.5 – 24.99
  - o Overweight: 25 – 29.99
  - o Obesity: >30
- Corpulence index: Height independent index
- Other criteria's for assessment of obesity:
  - o Ponderal index
  - o Lorentz formula
  - o Skin fold thickness
  - o Waist circumference & WHR/ Waist to hip ratio
- Abdominal fat accumulation is assessed by: Waist/ hip ratio
- WHR >0.85 in women suggest obesity
- WHR >1 in men suggest obesity

Ischemic/ Coronary Heart Disease:

- Known as modern epidemic
- Modifiable risk factors:
  - o Smoking
  - o High blood pressure
  - o Diabetes
  - o Raised cholesterol (>200 mg/ dl)
  - o Lack of exercise
- Non-Modifiable risk factors:
  - o Age
  - o Gender
  - o Positive family history
- Recommendations:
  - o Avoid alcohol consumption
  - o Reduce salt intake
  - o Promote complex carbohydrate consumption in diet

- o Limitation of dietary cholesterol
- o Reduction of fat intake

XII. OCCUPATIONAL DISEASES

Factory Act - 1948

- Maximum working hours of 48 hours/ week and if overtime, then 60 hours/ week
- Children less than 14 years should not be employed

Asbestosis:

- Exposure to: Asbestos dust
- Affects: Base of lungs
- Predisposes to:
  - o Mesothelioma
  - o Bronchogenic cancer
  - o Interstitial fibrosis (Ferruginous body)
  - o Pleural plaque

Bagassosis:

- Inhalation of sugar cane dust/ molasses/ fibrous residue of sugarcane (bagasse)
- Bagasse blocks bronchioles leading to bronchitis and bronchopneumonia
- Bagassosis is a form of extrinsic allergic alveolitis
- Prevention by 2% Propionic acid
- Thermoactinomyces saccharii causes: Bagassosis

Farmers lung:

- Organism causing Farmers lung: Micropolyspora faeni, Aspergillus fumigates
- Exposure to: Mouldy hay, grain, Straw

Byssinosis:

- Textile industry (cotton fibre)
- Monday fever is associated with: Byssinosis

Silicosis:

- Most common chronic occupational disorder
- Notifiable condition under: Factories Act,1948 and Mines Act, 1952
- Occupation associated with silicosis: Silica dust, mines, tunnels
- 0.5 – 3 micron size are particles are most dangerous
- Affects upper lobe of lung
- Chest X-ray shows egg shell calcification
- No effective treatment.
- Patient with silicosis are prone to develop:
  - o TB (silicotuberculosis) and nodular fibrosis,
  - o Emphysema and
  - o Cor pulmonale/ right sided heart failure
- Polarizing microscopy demonstrates birefringent crystals of silica.
- Snow storm appearance is seen in: Silicosis

ESI/ Employees State Insurance Act - 1948

- Covers:
  - o All non-power using factories with a minimum of 20 employees
  - o All power using factories with a minimum of 10 employees
- Chairman of ESI Corporation: Union minister of Labour
- Employees get: Full medical treatment for FREE
- Sickness benefit for employees:
  - o 50% of the average daily wages (for 91 days)
  - o Extended sickness benefit: Payable for 2 years for some specified diseases
  - o Enhanced sickness benefit: For vasectomy & tubectomy

XIII. BIOMEDICAL WASTE MANAGEMENT

COLOURED CONTAINERS, WASTE CATEGORIES & MODE OF TREATMENT

Red colour container:

- Contaminated waste (recyclable)
- Waste generated from disposable items such as tubing, bottles intravenous tubes

and sets, catheters, urine bags, syringes (without needles and fixed needle syringes) and vacutainers with their needles cut and gloves

- Treated by:
  - o Autoclaving/ chemical treatment/ microwaving

Yellow colour container:

- Human anatomical waste
- Animal anatomical waste
- Soiled waste
- Expired or discarded medicines
- Chemical wastes
- Chemical liquid waste
- Discarded linen, mattresses, beddings contaminated with blood or body fluids
- Microbiology, biotechnology and other clinical laboratory waste
- Treated by:
  - o Incineration, deep burial

Blue coloured container:

- Glasswares (broken or discarded and contaminated glass including medicine vials and ampoules except those contaminated with cytotoxic waste)
- Metallic body implants
- Treated by:
  - o Autoclaving/ microwaving/ shredding/ chemical treatment and destruction

White coloured container:

- Waste sharps including metals (needles, syringes with fixed needles, needles from needle tip cutter or burner, scalpels, blades or any other contaminated sharp object that may cause puncture and cutes)
- Treated by:
  - o Autoclaving or dry heat sterilization followed by shredding, mutilation or encapsulization in metallic containers or cement concrete

CATEGORIES OF BIO-MEDICAL WASTE

Category	*Biomedical waste*	*Includes:*
1	Human anatomical waste	Human tissues, body parts, organs, placenta
2	Animal waste	Animal tissues, body parts, organs, blood, carcasses, fluids
3	Microbiological and Biotechnology waste	Waste from laboratory cultures, human and animal cell culture used in research, waste from production of biological, toxins, dishes used for transfer of cultures
4	Waste sharp	Needles, scalpels, syringes, blade, glass
5	Discarded medicine and cytotoxic drugs	Waste comprising of outdated, conta-minated and discarded medicines
6	Soiled waste	Items contaminated with blood, and body fluids
7	Solid waste	Waste generated from disposal items other than sharp such as tubings, catheters, intravenous sets etc.
8	Liquid waste	Waste generated from laboratory and washing, cleaning, housekeeping etc.
9	Incineration ash	Ash generated from incineration of any biomedical waste
10	Chemical waste	Chemical used in production of biologicals or disinfection

XIV. HEALTH PLANNING

Chaddah committee:

- NMEP with general health services and Basic health worker per 10,000 population (for malaria vigilance, collection of vital statistics and family planning)

Kartar singh committee:

- MPHW under Health & family planning (ANMs to be replaced by 'Female Health Workers' and Basic health workers, Malaria surveillance workers, vaccinators, health education assistants to be replaced by 'Male Health Workers')

Bhore committee

- Health survey and development committee
- PHC/ primary health centre concept (1 PHC per 40,000 population, 30 beds, 3 subcenters and 2 medical officers),
- 3 months training in PSM (prepare social physicians)

XV. EPIDEMIOLOGY

TYPES OF STUDIES

Experimental studies:

- Randomized controlled trials
- Community trial
- Field trial

Observational studies:

- Descriptive
- Analytical
  - o Case control
  - o Cohort
  - o Cross-sectional
  - o Ecological

Case control study/ retrospective study:

- Suitable for: Rare diseases
- Backward looking study
- Effect to cause study
- Disease to risk factor study
- Outcome to cause study
- Rapid
- Easy
- Inexpensive
- No risk to subjects
- Multiple exposures can be checked
- No loss of follow-up
- Requires few subjects
- Cannot measure incidence
- Recall bias is a problem
- Case and control selection troublesome
- Yields: Odd's ratio

Cohort study/ prospective study:

- Reserved for testing of precisely formulated hypothesis
- Best way to identify incidence, natural history of a disease & can be used to examine multiple outcomes after a single exposure
- Forward looking study
- Cause to effect study
- Risk factor to disease study
- Exposure to outcome study
- Follow-up study
- Can examine rare exposures
- Can establish population based incidence
- Time-to-event analysis is possible
- Decreased selection and information bias
- Sampling & observer bias
- Loss to follow-up, migration or non-response bias
- Not suitable for conditions with long latency
- Not suitable for rare diseases
- Lengthy and expensive study
- Yields:
  - o Attributable risk,
  - o Relative risk
  - o Incidence

Strength of association:

	Disease	Non-diseased
Exposure	A	b
Non-exposed	C	d

Calculations:

- Odd's ratio (ad/bc)
  - o If Odd's ratio is more than 1, it signifies that exposure is a risk factor for disease and vice versa.
- Relative risk:

<u>Incidence of disease in exposed</u>
Incidence of disease in non-exposed
a/ a+b
c/ c+d

- If Relative risk is more than 1, it indicates exposure is a risk factor for disease (increases risk of disease) and vice-versa

Blind study:

- In single blind study, patient is not aware whether he is in the control or study group
- Double blind study:
  - o Patient does not know which treatment they are receiving
  - o Investigator/doctor does not know which treatment they are giving
- In triple blinding, along with patient and doctor, the person analyzing the data is also unaware/ blind

Tip of iceberg phenomenon:

- Bottom of iceberg: Subclinical cases of the disease
- Water-line: Differentiation between apparent and in apparent disease
- Submerged part: Undiagnosed cases in community (latent, presymptomatic cases)
- Floating tip: Clinical cases

Tools of measurement in epidemiology

- Number of new cases occurring during a specified time in a defined population, initially free of disease: Incidence
- Incidence = Prevalence/ average duration of the disease
- All cases counted on a single survey or examination of a group: Prevalence
- Occurrence of more cases of a disease than expected in a given area over a particular period of time: Epidemic
- Constant presence of a disease in a defined geographical area: Endemic
- Disease affecting a large geographical area such as part of a nation, continent or world: Pandemic
- Number of infant deaths per thousand live births: Infant Mortality Rate
- Number of maternal deaths per lakh live births: Maternal mortality Rate
- Number of exposed person's developing the disease within the range of the incubation period following exposure to primary cause: Secondary attack rate
- Time interval between receipt of infection & maximal infectivity: Generation time
- Period between diagnosis by early detection/ screening & diagnosis by other (routine) means: Lead time
- Gap between onset of primary case (1st case introduced) & secondary case (develops from primary case): Serial interval
- Number of deaths per 100 cases: Case fatality rate

Screening:

- True positive (sensitivity):
  - o A positive result in the presence of the disease
  - o Ability of screening test to identify correctly all those who have the disease
- True negative (Specificity):
  - o A negative test, in the absence of the disease
  - o Ability of screening test to identify correctly all those who do not have the disease
- Negative predictive value: Ability of a screening test to identify correctly all those who do not have the disease, out of all those who test negative on a screening test
- Positive predictive value: Ability of a screening test to identify correctly all those who have the disease, out of all those who test positive on a screening test

Disease:

- Control: Disease agent is allowed to persist in the community at a level where it ceases to be a public health problem.

- Eradication: Termination of all transmission of infection by extermination of the infectious agent
- Elimination: Intermediate goal between disease control and disease elimination

Surveillance:

- The continuous scrutiny of the risk factors that determine the occurrence and distribution of the disease
- Sentinel surveillance: A method for identifying the missing cases & thereby supplementing the notified cases

XVI. CONCEPTS OF HEALTH

Levels of prevention:

- Defluoridation of water/ provision of safe water & housing: Primary prevention
- Pap smear: Secondary prevention
- Salt restriction in non-communicable disease: Primordial prevention
- Cessation of smoking: Primordial prevention
- Immunization: Primary prevention
- IOL implantation (treatment) in cataract surgery: Secondary prevention
- Physiotherapy in a case with poliomyelitis: Tertiary prevention

Primordial prevention:

- Prevention of the emergence of the risk factors: Primordial prevention
- Best applied for chronic diseases, coronary artery disease, hypertension (non-communicable)
- Avoidance of smoking & fatty diet
- Exercise to avoid risk of CHD/ HTN
- Source reduction in malaria

Primary prevention:

- Action taken prior to onset of disease (health promotion & specific protection-immunization, chemoprophylaxis): Primary prevention
- Best applied for Vaccine preventable diseases
- The action is taken prior to onset of disease (risk factor present)
- Mode of intervention:
  - o Health promotion
  - o Specific protection
- Health promotion:
  - o Health education
  - o Lifestyle & behavioural change
  - o Nutritional intervention (food fortification)
  - o Environmental (safe water & housing)
- Specific protection:
  - o Immunization against VPDs
  - o Vitamin A prophylaxis
  - o Contraception for STDs
  - o Chemoprophylaxis
  - o Protection against occupational hazards, accidents, carcinogens & allergens
  - o Bed nets
  - o Quarantine

Secondary prevention:

- Action halting the progress of disease at early stage (early diagnosis & treatment): Secondary prevention
- Best applied for TB, leprosy, STDs
- Screening test & case finding (pap smear for Ca cervix)
- Treatment of TB, leprosy & STDs
- Its purpose is to cure disease, slow its progression or reduce its impact on individuals or communities

Tertiary prevention:

- Disability limitation & Rehabilitation: Tertiary prevention
- Best applied for polio
- Tertiary prevention strategies involve both therapeutic and rehabilitative measures once disease is firmly established

Must know terms:

- Provision of free medical services to people at GOVERNMENT expenses: State medicine

- Provision of medical services & professional education by STATE, but the programme is operated & regulated by PROFESSIONAL GROUPS rather than government: Socialized medicine
- Any loss/ abnormality of psychological, physiologic or anatomical structure or function (e.g. loss of foot, defective vision): Impairment
- Because of impairment, affected person may be unable to carry out certain activities, which may be considered normal for his age, sex (cannot walk): Disability

Indices:

- Infant mortality rate, Life expectancy at ONE year, Literacy rate:
  - o Physical Quality of Life Index/ PQLI
  - o Ranges from 0-100
- Expectation of life free of disability: Sullivan's index
- Burden of disease & effectiveness of interventions/ Years of life lost to premature death:
  - o Disability Adjusted Life Year/ DALY
  - o Highest DALY is for psychiatric disorders (Schizophrenia, unipolar/ bipolar disorders)
- Education, Occupation, Income: Kuppuswamy's index

XVII. DEMOGRAPHY & HEALTH

Demographic cycle:

Crude death rate	*Crude birth rate*	*Phase*	*Stage*
High	High	High stationary	I
Starts declining	High	Early expanding	II
Continue declining	Starts declining	Late expanding	III
Low	Low	Low stationary	IV
High	Low	Declining	V

Other indicators:

- Crude death rate: Total number of deaths in a year/ 1000 MYP (mid-year population)
- Crude birth rate: Total number of live birth in a year/ 1000 MYP
- Dependents age group: Above 65 years & below 15 years

XVIII. PSM IN OBSTETRICS & PPEDIATRICS

Fertility indicators:

- Net reproduction rate: Number of daughters a newborn girl will bear during her entire life time assuming fixed age specific fertility and mortality rates
- Gross reproduction rate: Number of daughters a newborn girl will bear during her entire life time if she experiences the current fertility throughout her reproductive age group assuming no mortality
- Total fertility rate: Average number of children a woman would bear in her reproductive age group (child-bearing age)
- General fertility rate: Number of live births per thousand women in the reproductive age group (15 to 45 years)

Intelligence quotient/ IQ:

- Calculated as: Mental age × 100/ Chronological age
- 0 - 25: Idiot
- 25 - 50: Imbecile
- 50 – 70: Moron
- 70 – 80: Borderline
- 80 – 90: Low normal
- 90 – 110: Normal
- 110 – 120: Superior
- 120 – 140: Very superior
- Above 140: Near Genius

Mental retardation:

- Mild: IQ of 50 – 70
- Moderate: IQ of 35 – 50
- Severe: IQ of 20 – 35
- Profound: IQ of less than 20